Introduction

Nutrition isn't just a routine; it's a lifeline. Imagine each meal as a chance to fuel your body, a moment to either support your health or put it at risk. This concept is more than theoretical—it's a guiding principle that can reshape how you view food and its role in your life.

Whole foods like—fruits, vegetables, whole grains, nuts, and legumes—pack in the nutrients your body craves. These foods provide vitamins, minerals, and antioxidants that combat oxidative stress and inflammation, fundamental contributors to chronic diseases. Eating a rainbow of colors on your plate ensures you're receiving a wide array of nutrients. The more colors, the better your chances of keeping your body functioning optimally. Consider the impact of nutrition on specific health outcomes. A well-rounded diet can help ward off conditions like obesity, diabetes, and heart disease. Research shows a direct correlation between diet and disease prevalence. High-fiber diets rich in whole grains and legumes help regulate blood sugar levels and lower cholesterol. Meanwhile, diets laden with processed foods and sugar can lead to metabolic disorders and increased inflammation. The choices you

How not to die:
Transform Your Health with Every Bite.

By David A. Owen phd

Table of contents

make at every meal matter immensely.

Transitioning to a nutrient-dense diet doesn't have to be overwhelming. Whether it's adding spinach to your morning smoothie or snacking on apple slices instead of chips, these small shifts can lead to big changes. Gradually, you can explore whole grains like quinoa, brown rice, and farro. Discovering plant-based proteins such as beans, lentils, and tofu will not only diversify your meals but also enhance your health.

Now, let's talk about the hidden dangers lurking in our diets. Processed foods often masquerade as healthy options. Something labeled "low-fat" may be loaded with sugar or artificial ingredients. Understanding food labels is crucial. Pay attention to the ingredients list. Aim for foods with fewer, recognizable components. When in doubt, choose whole foods that don't require a label.

The relationship between food and health extends beyond physical well-being. Diets rich in omega-3 fatty acids can bolster mood and cognitive function. Likewise, B vitamins found in leafy greens and whole grains support brain health. When you nourish your body with wholesome foods, you foster a better mental state as well.

Incorporating more plant-based meals into your diet offers substantial benefits. A plant-rich diet isn't just beneficial for your health; it's also linked to environmental sustainability. Reducing meat consumption can lessen your carbon footprint and promote the ethical treatment of animals. Start slow—try one meatless day a week. Explore new recipes that highlight vegetables as the centerpiece, rather than an afterthought.

Hydration often gets sidelined in discussions about nutrition, yet it's vital. Aim to drink water throughout the day, and incorporate hydrating foods like cucumbers, oranges, and watermelon. Cut down on sugary drinks, which can lead to weight gain and metabolic issues.

Learning to prepare your meals can transform your relationship with food. Basic cooking skills open up a world of possibilities. Start with simple techniques like steaming or roasting vegetables. As you grow more comfortable, experiment with herbs and spices to enhance flavor without extra calories. Engaging with cooking can be a rewarding experience that not only nourishes your body but also sparks joy in the kitchen. Mindful eating deserves attention. This practice involves tuning in to your body's hunger and fullness cues. Instead of eating mindlessly while scrolling through your phone, focus on the flavors and textures of your food. Savor each bite. This awareness not only enhances your enjoyment but also helps prevent overeating. When you pay attention to what you eat, you may discover that you're satisfied with less.

The importance of community cannot be overstated. Join forces with friends or family who share your health goals. Cooking together or sharing recipes can provide motivation and make healthy eating more enjoyable. Participating in local farmers' markets can foster a sense of community while encouraging healthier choices. Surround yourself with like-minded individuals who inspire you to embrace a healthier lifestyle.

Regular physical activity complements a healthy diet, creating a powerful synergy for overall well-being. Engage in activities you love, whether it's dancing, hiking, or yoga. Find ways to incorporate movement into your daily routine, like taking the stairs or going for a walk during your lunch break.

Every small change contributes to a healthier lifestyle. Don't feel pressured to overhaul your diet overnight. Focus on gradual shifts. Aim to include a fruit or vegetable with each meal. Discover new recipes that excite you. The journey toward better health is a process; celebrate each step you take, no matter how small.

The Foundations of Nutrition

Macronutrients Explained

Macronutrients are the big players in our diet. They include carbohydrates, proteins, and fats. Each one plays a unique role in our body. Carbohydrates are our main energy source. Proteins are the building blocks. They help repair tissues and build muscles. Fats, often misunderstood, are essential. They support cell growth, protect organs, and keep us warm.

Carbs come in two forms: simple and complex. Simple carbs are quick energy but can spike blood sugar. Proteins are found in meat, beans, and nuts. They're crucial for growth and repair. Fats are divided into saturated, unsaturated, and trans fats. Unsaturated fats, found in fish and olive oil, are the healthiest.

The Power of Micronutrients

Micronutrients, though needed in smaller amounts, are vital. They include vitamins and minerals. Some of the antioxidants are Vitamins like A, C, and E. They protect our cells from damage. B vitamins help convert food into energy. Minerals like calcium and iron are crucial. Calcium strengthens bones. Iron is essential for blood production.

Vitamins are either water-soluble or fat-soluble. Water-soluble vitamins, like C and B-complex, need regular replenishment. Fat-soluble vitamins, like A, D, E, and K, are stored in the body. Minerals are categorized into macro and trace minerals. Trace minerals, like zinc and selenium, are needed in smaller amounts but are equally important.

Understanding Dietary Fiber

It's found in plants. Fiber is crucial for digestive health. It aids in controlling how the body utilizes sugar, managing both hunger and blood sugar levels. Fiber comes in two forms: soluble and insoluble. Soluble fiber dissolves in water. Insoluble fiber doesn't dissolve in water. It helps food move through the digestive system, promoting regularity.

Fiber also helps maintain a healthy weight. It adds bulk to

the diet, making you feel full faster. This can help prevent overeating.

Balancing Your Plate

A balanced plate includes a variety of foods. Half your plate should be fruits and vegetables. They provide essential vitamins, minerals, and fiber. This can be meat, fish, beans, or nuts. The remaining quarter should be whole grains. These provide energy and fiber. Don't forget healthy fats.

Eating a variety of foods ensures you get all the nutrients you need. It's also important to stay hydrated. Water is essential for all bodily functions. Reduce the intake of sugary drinks and go for water or herbal teas. Balance is key. Enjoy treats in moderation.

Creating a balanced meal plan can be straightforward and enjoyable!

1. Set Your Health Goals

When you have your meal plan, you determine what you want to achieve.

2. Calculate Your Daily Caloric Needs

Use an online calculator to estimate your daily caloric needs based on your age, gender, weight, height, and activity level.

3. Include a Variety of Foods

Vegetables and fruit: Aim to fill half your plate with fruits and vegetables. They are rich in vitamins, minerals, and fiber.

Whole Grains: Opt for whole grains like brown rice, quinoa, and whole wheat bread. They provide sustained energy and fiber.

4. Plan Your Meals and Snacks

Breakfast: Combine protein, whole grains, and fruits. For example, oatmeal with berries and a side of Greek yogurt.

Lunch: Include lean protein, whole grain, and plenty of vegetables. A quinoa salad with grilled chicken and mixed greens works well.

Snacks: Choose healthy options like nuts, fruit, or hummus with veggies.

5. Create a Grocery list:

List all the ingredients required for your meal and snacks. This keeps you organized and ensures you have everything on hand.

6. Plan in advance:

Get your ingredients ready beforehand to save time throughout the week. Dice vegetables, cook grains, and divide snacks into portions.

7. Stay adaptable

Build some flexibility into your meal plan. Feel free to change meals or modify portions according to your appetite and schedule.

Sample Balanced Meal Plan

Day 1:

- Breakfast: Scrambled eggs with spinach and whole grain toast.

- Snack: Apple slices with almond butter.

Lunch: salad with grilled chicken, mixed with greens, cherry tomatoes and vinaigrette

Snacks: Greek yogurt topped with a few berries.

- Dinner: Baked salmon with quinoa and steamed broccoli.

Day 2:

-Breakfast: A smoothie made with banana, spinach, protein powder and almond milk.
- Snack: Carrot sticks with hummus.
- Lunch: whole grain tortilla wrap filled with turkey and avocado.
- Snack: Cottage cheese with pineapple chunks.
- Dinner: sautéed tofu with bell peppers, snap peas, and brown rice.

Tips for Success

-Diversity is essential: change up your fruits, Vegetables, protein and grain to maintain engaging and nutritious meals.
- stay hydrated: ensure you drink enough water daily, herbal tea and flavored water are also excellent choices.
- Listen to Your Body: Adjust portion sizes and meal frequency based on your hunger and energy levels.

Fruits and Vegetables

Carrot Sticks with Hummus: Crunchy and satisfying, with a boost of protein from the hummus.

Celery Sticks with Cream Cheese: A low-carb option that's creamy and filling.
Bell Pepper Slices with Guacamole: Packed with antioxidants and healthy fats.
Protein-Packed Snacks
Cottage Cheese with Pineapple: A sweet and savory mix that's rich in protein.
Nuts and Seeds
Mixed Nuts: A handful of nuts provides healthy fats, protein, and fiber.
Trail Mix: Combine nuts, seeds, and a few dark chocolate chips for a sweet and salty treat.
Whole Grains
1. Air-Popped Popcorn: A whole grain that's low in calories and high in fiber.
2. Whole Grain Crackers with Cheese: A balanced snack with carbs and protein.
3. Oatmeal with Fruit: A warm and comforting snack that's rich in fiber.
Smoothies
2. Berry Smoothie: Mix berries, Greek yogurt, and a splash of orange juice.
Other Healthy Options

1 . Dark Chocolate: A small piece of dark chocolate can satisfy your sweet tooth while providing antioxidants.

2. Rice Cakes with Avocado: Top rice cakes with mashed avocado and a sprinkle of salt.

3. Energy Balls: Made with oats, nut butter, and a bit of honey, these are perfect for a quick energy boost.

The Impact of Processed Foods

Processed foods dominate the modern diet. They appear in various forms: canned goods, frozen meals, snacks, and even seemingly healthy options like granola bars. But what exactly are processed foods? Essentially, they are any foods that have been altered from their original state. This alteration can involve adding ingredients, such as sugar, salt, and fats, or removing elements, like fiber and nutrients. While some processing is harmless, such as freezing vegetables, many processed foods come with significant health risks.

What Are Processed Foods?

At their core, processed foods fall into several categories based on their level of processing. Unprocessed or minimally processed foods include fresh fruits, vegetables, and nuts. These foods maintain their natural state, offering essential nutrients without additives. On the other hand, ultra-processed foods take a different route. They often contain ingredients you wouldn't find in your kitchen—preservatives, artificial flavors, and sweeteners. Items like sugary cereals, ready-to-eat meals, and sugary drinks exemplify this category.

Why does this distinction matter? Because the more food is processed, the more it tends to lose nutritional value. Whole foods retain vitamins, minerals, and fiber, while ultra-processed options often replace these benefits with empty calories. Eating these foods can lead to nutrient deficiencies, affecting overall health.

Health Risks Associated with Processed Foods

The health risks linked to processed foods are well-documented and alarming. Research shows that a diet high in processed foods correlates with numerous health issues. One major concern is obesity. Processed foods often contain high levels of sugar and unhealthy fats, making them calorie-dense but nutrient-poor. This combination can lead to weight gain and, ultimately, obesity.

Obesity is not just a cosmetic issue; it's a gateway to chronic diseases. Conditions like type 2 diabetes, heart disease, and certain cancers have all been tied to excessive processed food consumption. For instance, studies reveal that consuming high levels of added sugars significantly increases the risk of heart disease. The body struggles to process these sugars efficiently, leading to insulin resistance and inflammation.

Moreover, processed foods can alter gut health. The microbiome, which plays a crucial role in digestion and immunity, thrives on fiber-rich foods. Processed foods typically lack this essential component. A diet high in these foods can lead to an imbalance in gut bacteria, which may contribute to gastrointestinal disorders and other health issues.

Additives in processed foods present another risk. Many of these items contain artificial ingredients, some of which have raised health concerns. For example, certain food colorings and preservatives have been linked to hyperactivity in children and other adverse reactions. Additionally, the long-term effects of consuming these substances remain uncertain.

Mental health also takes a hit with processed food consumption. Studies indicate a connection between diets rich in ultra-processed foods and higher rates of depression and anxiety. The exact reasons for this correlation are still being explored, but the impact of poor nutrition on brain health cannot be ignored. Nutrient deficiencies, inflammation, and gut health all play a role in mental well-being.

Reading Food Labels

Navigating the grocery store can be daunting, especially when trying to make healthier choices. Food labels serve as essential guides. They provide valuable information about what you're putting into your body, but they can also be misleading.

Start with the ingredient list. The first few items reveal the main components of the product. If sugar appears among the first three ingredients, consider putting it back on the shelf. Watch out for various names of sugar, including high-fructose corn syrup, sucrose, and cane syrup. These hidden sugars contribute to the overall sugar content, increasing the risk of health issues.

Next, look at the nutrition facts panel. Pay attention to serving sizes, as they can be deceiving. A bag of chips might seem small, but a single serving could be just a handful, leading to mindless overeating. Examine calories per serving and the amounts of saturated fat, trans fat, and sodium. High levels of these components raise the risk of heart disease and hypertension.

Fiber content is a crucial factor. A good rule of thumb is to aim for products with at least three grams of fiber per serving. Fiber aids digestion and promotes satiety, helping to control hunger.

Lastly, keep an eye on health claims. A product labeled "low fat" may compensate with added sugars. "Natural" doesn't necessarily mean healthy, as processed foods can still carry this label. Scrutinize the ingredients rather than relying solely on marketing.

Choosing Whole Foods Instead

Embracing whole foods is a powerful way to enhance health and well-being. Whole foods are those that undergo minimal processing, preserving their natural state and nutritional integrity. Fruits, vegetables, legumes, whole grains, nuts, and seeds all fall into this category.

Leafy greens, berries, and cruciferous vegetables, such as broccoli and cauliflower, offer exceptional health benefits.

Whole grains are another excellent addition. Unlike refined grains, whole grains retain their fiber and nutrients. Foods like brown rice, quinoa, and oats are nutrient-dense choices. They not only support digestive health but also provide sustained energy, keeping you fuller for longer.

Legumes, including beans, lentils, and chickpeas, are powerhouse foods. Packed with protein, fiber, and essential vitamins, they serve as excellent meat alternatives. Incorporating legumes into your diet can help reduce reliance on processed proteins, like deli meats and pre-packaged meals.

Nuts and seeds offer healthy fats and essential nutrients. Snack on almonds, walnuts, or pumpkin seeds, or add them to salads and smoothies. These foods provide satiety and a wealth of vitamins and minerals.

Planning meals around whole foods can also save money. Fresh produce, grains, and legumes are often more affordable than packaged items. Preparing meals at home allows for greater control over ingredients, promoting healthier eating habits.

To transition toward whole foods, start small. As you become accustomed to these changes, explore new recipes and cooking methods. Simple meals can be delicious and nutritious.

Incorporating whole foods into your diet does not mean sacrificing flavor. Herbs and spices can enhance meals without adding calories or harmful ingredients. Experiment with different combinations to discover new favorites.

Ultimately, embracing whole foods can transform health. Reducing processed food intake helps mitigate risks associated with obesity, chronic diseases, and mental health issues. By making informed choices, you empower yourself to cultivate a healthier lifestyle.

In a world overflowing with processed options, choosing whole foods is a radical act of self-care. It requires mindfulness, effort, and a willingness to prioritize well-being. As awareness grows regarding the impact of processed foods, many are reclaiming their health through mindful eating.

With each meal, consider the food's origin. How was it processed? What ingredients were used? By shifting focus from convenience to nourishment, individuals can foster a deeper connection to their food, leading to improved health and a more vibrant life.

Antioxidants: Your Body's Defense

Antioxidants play a vital role in maintaining health. They act as protectors against oxidative stress, a process where harmful molecules called free radicals damage cells. Understanding antioxidants and their benefits is crucial for anyone aiming to improve their health and longevity.

What Are Antioxidants?

Antioxidants are naturally occurring substances found in many foods. Their primary function is to neutralize free radicals—unstable molecules that can cause cellular damage. Free radicals form from various sources, including environmental pollutants, UV radiation, and even normal metabolic processes. The body constantly battles these free radicals, and antioxidants provide a crucial line of defense.

Vitamins like C and E, minerals like selenium, and a host of phytochemicals all serve as antioxidants. Each type works differently, but their goal remains the same: to protect cells from oxidative damage. When the balance tips toward more free radicals than antioxidants, oxidative stress occurs, leading to inflammation, cellular aging, and the development of chronic conditions such as heart disease, cancer, and neurodegenerative disorders.

Understanding how antioxidants work is essential. When free radicals are present, they seek to stabilize themselves by stealing electrons from nearby molecules. This process can cause a chain reaction, damaging proteins, lipids, and DNA in the process. Antioxidants step in to donate electrons without becoming destabilized themselves. This unique ability allows them to interrupt the cycle of damage.

Different antioxidants serve different functions. For example, vitamin C primarily protects the aqueous (water-filled) compartments of the body, such as blood and tissues, while vitamin E protects fatty areas, like cell membranes. Some antioxidants, like flavonoids, offer additional benefits by supporting the immune system and reducing inflammation. The diversity of antioxidants in the diet helps ensure comprehensive protection against oxidative stress.

Top Antioxidant-Rich Foods

Incorporating a variety of antioxidant-rich foods into your diet can enhance overall health. Below are some of the most potent sources of Berries: Blueberries, strawberries, raspberries, and blackberries rank high on the antioxidant scale. These fruits contain anthocyanins, powerful compounds linked to reduced inflammation and improved brain health. A handful of berries can provide a significant antioxidant boost.

Dark Leafy Greens: Vegetables like spinach, kale, and Swiss chard are packed with vitamins A, C, and K, as well as various phytonutrients. These greens not only combat oxidative stress but also support overall bodily functions, including bone health and vision.

Nuts: Walnuts, pecans, and almonds are rich in vitamin E and healthy fats. A small serving can provide a substantial amount of antioxidants. Nuts also contribute to heart health, making them an excellent snack choice.

Beans: Legumes, particularly black beans and kidney beans, boast high levels of antioxidants. They are also excellent sources of protein and fiber, promoting satiety and supporting digestive health.

Herbs and Spices: Many herbs and spices are antioxidant powerhouses. Turmeric, for instance, contains curcumin, known for its anti-inflammatory properties. Other herbs, such as oregano and cinnamon, also pack a significant antioxidant punch.

Cruciferous Vegetables: Broccoli, Brussels sprouts, and cauliflower contain glucosinolates, compounds that provide antioxidant effects and support liver detoxification. Regular consumption of these vegetables may contribute to reduced cancer risk.

Whole Grains: Foods like oats, quinoa, and brown rice provide antioxidants along with fiber and essential nutrients. Whole grains promote digestive health and help regulate blood sugar levels.

Dark Chocolate: Good news for chocolate lovers! Dark chocolate, with a high cocoa content, contains flavonoids that exhibit antioxidant properties. Consuming it in moderation can offer health benefits while satisfying a sweet tooth.

Fruits: Beyond berries, other fruits like oranges, cherries, and grapes are rich in vitamins and phytochemicals. Citrus fruits, in particular, offer a substantial dose of vitamin C, a key player in the antioxidant defense system.

The goal is to create a colorful plate filled with various foods. Different colors represent different antioxidants, each providing unique health benefits. A diverse diet ensures that you receive a broad spectrum of protective compounds.

How Antioxidants Combat Aging

Aging affects everyone, but how we age can be influenced by our dietary choices. By combating oxidative stress, they help maintain cellular integrity and function.

One of the most significant effects of oxidative damage is its contribution to the aging of the skin. Free radicals can degrade collagen and elastin, proteins essential for skin elasticity and firmness. As antioxidants neutralize free radicals, they help protect these proteins, keeping skin healthier for longer.

Additionally, antioxidants support brain health. Aging can lead to cognitive decline, but a diet rich in antioxidants may slow this process. Studies indicate that antioxidants, particularly those found in berries, can enhance memory and cognitive function. They reduce inflammation in the brain, which is often linked to neurodegenerative diseases like Alzheimer's.

Antioxidants also play a role in heart health. By preventing oxidative stress, they help maintain the integrity of blood vessels and reduce inflammation. Regular consumption of antioxidant-rich foods can improve cholesterol levels and lower blood pressure, promoting heart health at one age.

Moreover, antioxidants can bolster the immune system. Aging often comes with a decline in immune function, making individuals more susceptible to infections. Antioxidants support immune cells, enhancing their ability to fight off pathogens. A robust immune system can make a significant difference in overall health and longevity.

Research continues to explore how antioxidants affect aging on a cellular level. Telomeres, the protective caps on the ends of chromosomes, shorten as we age, leading to cellular aging. Some studies suggest that antioxidants may help preserve telomere length, contributing to cellular longevity.

While antioxidants have immense benefits, balance is key. Relying solely on supplements can be misleading and may not provide the same protective effects as whole foods. Whole foods contain a complex mixture of nutrients that work synergistically, providing enhanced benefits beyond isolated antioxidants.

Incorporating Antioxidants into Your Diet

Making dietary changes to include more antioxidants doesn't have to be overwhelming. Start by making simple swaps and gradually incorporating more antioxidant-rich foods into meals.

Begin your day with a smoothie. Toss in a handful of spinach or kale, add some berries, and blend with almond milk. This combination packs a powerful antioxidant punch to kickstart your morning. You can also add a tablespoon of flaxseeds or chia seeds for extra fiber and omega-3 fatty acids.

For lunch, create a vibrant salad. Use dark leafy greens as a base and top with various colorful vegetables—think tomatoes, bell peppers, and carrots. Add a handful of nuts or seeds for crunch and sprinkle some herbs for flavor. A drizzle of olive oil and lemon juice completes the dish while providing healthy fats. Snack smartly by opting for fruits or nuts instead of processed snacks. Keep berries on hand for a quick, nutritious treat. Alternatively, choose apple slices with almond butter or a handful of walnuts. These choices not only satisfy hunger but also contribute to your antioxidant intake.

Incorporating beans into meals is simple. Add them to soups, stews, or salads. They provide protein, fiber, and antioxidants. A hearty black bean chili can be both comforting and nutrient-dense.

When cooking, explore the world of herbs and spices. Use turmeric in curries or cinnamon in oatmeal. These ingredients not only add flavor but also enhance the antioxidant content of your meals.

For dinner, focus on colorful vegetables. Roast a medley of broccoli, carrots, and Brussels sprouts tossed in olive oil. Pair with a whole grain like quinoa or brown rice for a complete meal. Incorporating a variety of vegetables ensures you benefit from a range of antioxidants.

Experiment with different recipes and cooking methods. Stir-frying, roasting, and grilling can bring out the natural flavors and nutrients in vegetables. Make sure there are enough vegetables on your plate whenever you are having your meal.

Don't forget about dessert. Opt for dark chocolate as a treat. A few squares can satisfy your sweet tooth while offering health benefits. Overall, the key lies in variety and balance. Aim for a colorful, diverse diet filled with whole foods. Each meal presents an opportunity to nourish your body with antioxidants. Prioritizing antioxidant-rich foods not only supports health but also enhances overall well-being. By making informed choices and being mindful of what you eat, you empower yourself to create a healthier lifestyle. Embrace the journey toward better nutrition, and enjoy the delicious foods that support your body's natural defenses.

The Anti-Inflammatory Diet

Inflammation often gets a bad rap. It's a natural response of the body's immune system, helping to protect against injury and infection. However, when Inflammation persists over time, it can result in various health problems, such as heart disease, diabetes and autoimmune disorders. Understanding inflammation, the foods that combat it, and how to integrate them into your diet can make a significant difference in your health.

Understanding Inflammation

When the body encounters harmful stimuli—like pathogens, damaged cells, or irritants—it reacts with inflammation. This process involves immune cells, blood vessels, and proteins working together to heal tissue and fight infections. You might notice this response as swelling, redness, or warmth in the affected area. For example, a sprained ankle swells as blood flows to the area to aid healing. This acute inflammation is beneficial.

Chronic inflammation, however, occurs when this response lingers longer than necessary. Instead of aiding healing, it starts damaging tissues. Factors like poor diet, lack of exercise, stress, and environmental toxins can contribute to this unwanted condition. Over time, chronic inflammation can promote diseases such as arthritis, cardiovascular disease, and even cancer.

The link between inflammation and health has become a focal point in research. Inflammation can affect the entire body, contributing to fatigue, digestive issues, and mood disorders. Knowing the signs of chronic inflammation—like persistent fatigue, joint pain, or digestive disturbances—can help individuals address it before it leads to more serious health concerns.

Inflammation also has a connection to the gut. The gut microbiome, the community of bacteria residing in the intestines, plays a critical role in regulating inflammation. An imbalance in gut bacteria can lead to increased inflammation and various health issues. Supporting gut health through diet can positively influence inflammation levels.

Foods That Fight Inflammation

Certain foods act as natural anti-inflammatories, providing the body with the tools it needs to combat chronic inflammation. Incorporating these foods into your diet can create a powerful defense system.

Fruits and Vegetables: Vibrant produce stands out for a reason. Berries—like blueberries, strawberries, and blackberries—are especially rich in anthocyanins, compounds known to reduce inflammation. Leafy greens, like spinach, kale, and Swiss chard are rich in nutrients and antioxidants that aid in fighting inflammation. Brightly colored vegetables, including carrots, bell peppers, and beets, also contribute beneficial compounds.

These foods are rich in omega-3 fatty acids, which possess powerful anti-inflammatory properties. Walnuts, in particular, stand out as a great source of plant-based omega-3s. Just a small handful can significantly impact inflammation levels.

These fish contain EPA and DHA, types of omega-3s that have been shown to reduce inflammation. Regular consumption can improve heart health and lower the risk of chronic diseases.

Whole Grains: Foods like brown rice, quinoa, oats, and barley are high in fiber, which plays a role in reducing inflammation. Fiber helps support a healthy gut microbiome, which in turn can lower inflammation levels. Whole grains also provide essential nutrients that the body needs to function optimally.

Legumes: Beans, lentils, and chickpeas are not only rich in protein and fiber, but they also contain a variety of phytochemicals that combat inflammation. Incorporating legumes into meals can enhance satiety while providing numerous health benefits.

Herbs and Spices: Many herbs and spices offer remarkable anti-inflammatory properties. Turmeric, for instance, contains curcumin, a potent compound that fights inflammation. Ginger, garlic, and cinnamon also possess beneficial effects. Adding these spices to dishes can elevate flavor while boosting health benefits.

Olive Oil: Extra virgin olive oil, a staple of the Mediterranean diet, is rich in healthy fats and antioxidants. Drizzling olive oil over salads or using it for cooking can provide both flavor and health benefits.

Dark Chocolate: High-quality dark chocolate, particularly varieties with at least 70% cocoa, contains flavonoids that may reduce inflammation. Consuming dark chocolate in moderation can satisfy a sweet tooth while providing health benefits.

Incorporating these foods into daily meals can create a powerful anti-inflammatory arsenal. Aim for variety, as different foods contribute different nutrients. A diverse diet ensures comprehensive protection against inflammation.

Meal Planning for Anti-Inflammation

Planning meals centered around anti-inflammatory foods can be straightforward and enjoyable. Start by stocking your kitchen with key ingredients. Having these items on hand makes it easier to whip up healthy meals.

Breakfast Ideas: Begin the day with a nutrient-packed smoothie. Blend spinach, banana, berries, and a tablespoon of flaxseeds for a delicious and filling breakfast. Sometimes overnight oats can also be a great option. Combine oats with almond milk, chia seeds, and fruit, letting it sit overnight for a quick, healthy breakfast.

Lunch Options: For lunch, consider a colorful salad filled with leafy greens, cherry tomatoes, bell peppers, and avocados. Top it with walnuts and a drizzle of olive oil for added flavor. A grain bowl with quinoa, black beans, roasted vegetables, and a sprinkle of turmeric can be both satisfying and nutritious.

Dinner Choices: Dinner can feature fatty fish like salmon, grilled and served with a side of steamed broccoli and quinoa. Stir-frying a mix of colorful vegetables with garlic and ginger, then serving it over brown rice, can create a vibrant and healthful meal.

Snacks: Keep healthy snacks handy. Fresh fruit, raw nuts, or vegetable sticks with hummus are excellent choices. Prepare energy bites made from oats, nut butter, and dark chocolate for a quick, nutritious treat.

Batch Cooking: Preparing meals in batches can save time and make it easier to stick to an anti-inflammatory diet. Cook a large pot of vegetable soup, chili, or grain salads that can be enjoyed throughout the week. This not only simplifies meal prep but ensures that healthy options are always available.

Exploring New Recipes: Experimenting with new recipes can keep meals exciting. Look for dishes that highlight anti-inflammatory ingredients. For instance, try a turmeric-infused lentil soup or a quinoa salad with roasted beets and walnuts.

Dining Out: When eating out, opt for dishes that focus on whole foods. Choose salads, grain bowls, and vegetable-heavy options. Meal planning requires creativity and intention. It can be helpful to set aside a few hours each week to plan meals, shop for ingredients, and prepare foods in advance. This not only promotes healthier eating but can also enhance overall well-being.

Lifestyle Changes to Reduce Inflammation

Diet alone isn't the only factor in combating inflammation. Adopting a holistic approach can amplify the benefits of an anti-inflammatory diet. Making lifestyle changes can create a supportive environment for reducing inflammation.

Regular Exercise: Physical activity plays a crucial role in managing inflammation. Engaging in moderate exercise, such as walking, swimming, or cycling, can help lower inflammatory markers in the body. Not only does exercise reduce inflammation, but it also improves mood and boosts overall health.

Stress Management: Chronic stress contributes to inflammation. Integrating stress-reduction techniques into your daily routine can be beneficial. Mindfulness activities like meditation and yoga encourage relaxation and lower stress levels. Spending time in nature, journaling, or engaging in hobbies can also serve as effective stress relievers.

Sufficient sleep is essential for overall well-being. Lack of sleep can raise inflammation levels in the body. Strive for 7 to 9 hours of restorative sleep each night.

Stay Hydrated: Drinking plenty of water supports overall health and aids in maintaining proper bodily functions. Aim to drink enough water throughout the day, and consider herbal teas, which can also provide anti-inflammatory benefits.

Avoiding Processed Foods: Reducing the intake of processed foods is crucial in managing inflammation. Emphasize whole, unprocessed food as the basis of your diet.

Limiting Sugar Intake: High sugar consumption can contribute to inflammation and various health issues. Read food labels to identify hidden sugars and aim to limit sugary beverages, desserts, and processed snacks.

Mindful Eating: Paying attention to what you eat can lead to better choices. This approach can help you appreciate food more and make conscious decisions about what you consume.

Social Connections: Maintaining social connections can support mental and emotional well-being. Surround yourself with supportive friends and family.

Regular Check-ups: Staying proactive about health is vital. Regular check-ups can help identify inflammation-related issues early. Work with a healthcare professional to monitor inflammatory markers and receive guidance on maintaining a healthy lifestyle.

By implementing these lifestyle changes alongside an anti-inflammatory diet, individuals can create a comprehensive strategy to combat inflammation. The journey toward better health may require effort and commitment, but the rewards are significant.

Embracing an anti-inflammatory diet and making a conscious lifestyle

Superfoods for SuperHealth

Defining Superfoods

Superfoods burst onto the scene, capturing attention for their impressive health benefits. These foods are nutrient powerhouses, packed with vitamins, minerals, antioxidants, and other compounds that promote health. While there's no official definition, superfoods generally refer to foods that offer significant health benefits, often beyond basic nutrition. They can help prevent disease, enhance well-being, and boost energy. Think of them as the elite athletes of the food world—concentrated sources of good that pack a punch.

Imagine biting into a blueberry. Not only is it delicious, but it's also rich in antioxidants that combat oxidative stress. Every bite contributes to heart health, brain function, and even skin vitality. Superfoods can range from fruits and vegetables to nuts, seeds, and grains. Their unique properties can improve your overall health when included in a balanced diet.

Top Superfoods Include

1. Blueberries Bursting with antioxidants, particularly anthocyanins, blueberries top the list. These tiny berries protect against oxidative damage, reduce inflammation, and support brain health. Toss them into smoothies, sprinkle them over oatmeal, or eat them by the handful for a tasty boost.

2. Kale A leafy green superstar, kale is loaded with vitamins A,

C, and K. Its fiber content aids digestion, while its antioxidants may lower the risk of chronic diseases. Use it in salads, or smoothies, or sauté it as a side dish for a nutrient-dense addition to any meal.

3. Quinoa This grain-like seed is a complete protein, containing all nine essential amino acids. Quinoa is also high in fiber and magnesium, making it a fantastic option for vegetarians and vegans. Use it as a base for salads, in stir-fries, or as a side dish to complement your favorite proteins.

4. Salmon Fatty fish like salmon provide omega-3 fatty acids, essential for heart and brain health. Grill it, bake it, or add it to salads for a satisfying and nutritious meal.

5. Chia Seeds Small but mighty, chia seeds are packed with fiber, protein, and omega-3 fatty acids. They absorb liquid, forming a gel-like consistency that helps keep you full. Mix them into smoothies, or yogurt, or make a chia pudding for a healthy snack.

6. Spinach Spinach boasts a rich array of vitamins and minerals,

including iron and calcium. Its antioxidants support eye health and reduce the risk of chronic diseases. Use fresh spinach in salads, blend it into smoothies, or sauté it for a quick side dish.

7. Sweet Potatoes A delicious source of complex carbohydrates, sweet potatoes are rich in beta-carotene, which converts to vitamin A in the body. Their high fiber content supports digestive health. Bake them, mash them, or add them to soups for a comforting, nutritious option.

8. Turmeric Known for its bright yellow color, turmeric contains curcumin, a powerful anti-inflammatory compound. This spice may help alleviate pain and support overall health. Incorporate it into

Gut Health and Nutrition

The gut microbiome is a bustling metropolis of microorganisms residing in your intestines. It consists of trillions of bacteria, fungi, viruses, and other microbes, all playing crucial roles in your health. This community is diverse; each person's microbiome is unique, and influenced by diet, environment, and lifestyle. Research has shown that a healthy gut microbiome can support digestion, enhance mood, and even influence chronic diseases.

Understanding the gut microbiome begins with recognizing its complexity. Microbes work together symbiotically, breaking down food particles and helping to extract nutrients. They help in the fermentation of dietary fibers, producing short-chain fatty acids that fuel intestinal cells and contribute to overall health. This collaboration between different species is essential for maintaining balance. When this balance is disrupted, dysbiosis occurs, leading to potential health issues such as inflammatory bowel disease, obesity, and diabetes.

Foods you consume directly influence which microbes thrive and which diminish. Diets rich in sugar and processed food may result in the excessive growth of harmful bacteria. Conversely, a diet rich in whole, plant-based foods promotes diversity and stability within the microbiome. The types of fibers consumed, for instance, can determine which beneficial bacteria flourish.

Foods That Promote Gut Health

Eating for gut health means prioritizing whole foods. Leafy greens, vegetables, fruits, legumes, nuts, and seeds contain fiber that supports beneficial bacteria. Fermented foods also deserve attention. Foods like yogurt, kefir, sauerkraut, kimchi, and kombucha provide probiotics, the live microorganisms that add to the population of good bacteria in your gut. These foods not only support digestion but also enhance the immune response and reduce inflammation.

Incorporating a variety of colors on your plate ensures a wide range of nutrients and phytochemicals. Each color often indicates different health benefits; for instance, orange and yellow fruits and vegetables are high in carotenoids, while dark leafy greens provide folate and vitamin K. Aim for diversity— different types of fiber feed different microbes, helping to maintain a robust microbiome.

Whole grains are another cornerstone of gut health. Foods like oats, brown rice, quinoa, and barley contain soluble fiber, which helps to regulate blood sugar levels and provides nourishment for beneficial bacteria. The fermentation process of these fibers produces substances that can lower cholesterol and improve gut barrier function.

Spices and herbs add not only flavor but also health benefits. Garlic, onions, leeks, and asparagus are prebiotic foods that feed healthy gut bacteria. Turmeric, containing the active ingredient curcumin, is recognized for its anti-inflammatory effect.

Nuts and seeds, particularly flaxseeds and chia seeds, offer omega-3 fatty acids and soluble fiber, promoting gut health. Aim for raw or lightly roasted varieties without added sugars or salts to maximize benefits.

The Link Between Gut Health and Immunity

The gut houses about 70% of the immune system. This relationship underscores the significance of maintaining gut health. A balanced microbiome supports an effective immune response. Beneficial bacteria produce substances that can fend off harmful pathogens, acting as a first line of defense. When the microbiome is disrupted, the risk of infections and autoimmune diseases increases.

Research indicates that gut health influences systemic inflammation. Chronic low-grade inflammation often stems from an imbalanced gut microbiome, leading to conditions such as allergies, asthma, and even some autoimmune disorders. Supporting gut health through diet can mitigate these risks. A healthy microbiome can also enhance the efficacy of vaccines by influencing how the body responds to them.

Moreover, certain microbes produce metabolites that directly impact immune cells. These metabolites can help regulate immune responses, enhancing the body's ability to fight infections while reducing excessive inflammation.

The gut-brain axis further illustrates the connection between gut health and overall wellness. Gut bacteria produce neurotransmitters and other signaling molecules that can influence mood and cognitive function. Imbalances in the microbiome may contribute to conditions like anxiety and depression, highlighting the importance of a healthy diet for mental health as well.

Probiotics and Prebiotics

Probiotics consist of live beneficial bacteria that can enhance or restore gut flora. Each strain of probiotics has different benefits. For example, Lactobacillus and Bifidobacterium are among the most studied strains and have been shown to support digestive health and enhance immunity.

When choosing probiotics, look for products with multiple strains and a high CFU (colony-forming unit) count. It's also important to consider the delivery method, as some probiotics may not survive stomach acid. Fermented foods naturally contain these beneficial bacteria, making them an excellent option for enhancing gut health.

Prebiotics are non-digestible fibers that nourish the beneficial bacteria in your gut. Foods high in probiotics are bananas, onion and garlic, asparagus and wholegrain. Incorporating these into your diet can help to increase the population of beneficial bacteria, promoting balance in the microbiome.

The interaction between probiotics and prebiotics is crucial for keeping the gut healthy. Probiotics bring in helpful bacteria, while prebiotics supply the nutrients necessary for the bacteria to grow and flourish. Together, they can enhance digestive health, improve nutrient absorption, and strengthen the immune system. Understanding the delicate balance of the gut microbiome empowers individuals to make informed dietary choices. Prioritizing whole, plant-based foods, incorporating fermented products, and being mindful of fiber intake can significantly impact gut health and, by extension, overall well-being.

The Effect of stress and lifestyle on digestive health

Stress and lifestyle choices also significantly affect gut health. Long-time stress can disturb the microbiome's balance, resulting in dysbiosis. Stress hormones can influence gut motility and permeability, contributing to conditions like irritable bowel syndrome (IBS). Mindful practices such as yoga, meditation, and regular exercise can help manage stress levels and, in turn, support gut health.

Sleep is another critical factor. Poor sleep quality can exacerbate gut issues and contribute to an unhealthy microbiome. Strive for 7 to 9 hours of good sleep every night. Maintaining a consistent sleep routine and setting up a camping environment can improve sleep quality.

Avoiding excessive alcohol and tobacco is also crucial for gut health. Both substances can negatively affect gut microbiota and compromise the gut barrier, leading to increased permeability, often referred to as "leaky gut." Limiting or eliminating these substances can contribute to a healthier microbiome.

Proper hydration is essential for digestion for overall gut health. Adequate water intake helps preserve the intestinal mucosal lining and aids in the digestive process. Aim for adequate fluid intake throughout the day, focusing on water and herbal teas.

The Role of Diet in Preventing Disease

Research increasingly highlights the role of diet in preventing chronic diseases linked to gut health. Conditions such as obesity, diabetes, and cardiovascular diseases have been associated with an unhealthy gut microbiome. A diet rich in fruits, vegetables, whole grains, and fermented foods can help reduce the risk of these conditions.

For instance, studies have shown that a plant-based diet can promote a healthier microbiome. These diets are typically higher in fiber and lower in unhealthy fats and sugars, fostering a more balanced gut environment. The anti-inflammatory properties of many plant-based foods can also play a significant role in disease prevention.

Incorporating foods with high antioxidant properties can also be beneficial. Berries, nuts, and green tea are examples of foods rich in antioxidants that help combat oxidative stress and inflammation. This can be particularly important for gut health, as inflammation can damage the gut lining and disrupt the microbiome.

Monitoring and adjusting dietary habits based on individual responses can be a powerful tool. Keeping a food diary to track foods that cause discomfort or inflammation can help tailor dietary choices to support gut health. This approach can empower individuals to make positive changes based on their own experiences.

Supplements for Gut Health

While whole foods should form the foundation of a gut-healthy diet, certain supplements can offer additional support. Probiotic supplements may be beneficial for individuals with specific gut health concerns. When selecting a probiotic, consider factors such as strain diversity and CFU count.

Prebiotic supplements, like inulin or fructooligosaccharides (FOS), can also support gut health.

These fibers promote the growth of beneficial bacteria and can be beneficial for individuals who may not get enough prebiotic-rich foods in their diet.

Digestive enzymes can assist in breaking down food, making nutrients more accessible. For those with digestive issues, enzyme supplements may improve nutrient absorption and reduce discomfort. However, it's essential to approach supplements with caution and prioritize a whole-food diet as the primary source of nutrients.

The Future of Gut Health Research

Research into gut health continues to evolve, revealing new insights into the complexities of the microbiome. Studies are exploring the relationship between the microbiome and mental health, the effects of specific dietary patterns, and the potential for personalized nutrition based on microbiome composition. As our understanding grows, so too does the potential for tailored dietary recommendations that promote optimal gut health.

Advancements in technology are also facilitating research in this field. The ability to analyze and sequence the gut microbiome is becoming more accessible, allowing for a better understanding of individual microbiome profiles. This information can lead to more personalized dietary and health strategies.

Incorporating gut health considerations into overall health and wellness will become increasingly important. Awareness of the gut's role in various health conditions is growing, highlighting the need for a comprehensive approach to health that considers the microbiome.

Ultimately, fostering a healthy gut is about creating a balanced lifestyle that prioritizes whole foods, stress management, quality sleep, and regular physical activity.

The Role of Hydration

Water makes up a large part of your body, about 60% of adults. From regulating temperature to facilitating digestion and nutrient absorption, water is essential. Your body continuously loses water through sweat, urine, and even breathing. To maintain optimal health, you need to replenish what you lose.

Water supports the functions of your organs. It aids the kidneys in filtering waste from your blood. If you don't drink enough, these organs can struggle, leading to issues. Your brain relies on hydration for clarity and focus. Studies show that even mild dehydration can affect mood and cognitive function. Keeping hydrated helps prevent headaches and fatigue, both of which can disrupt daily life.

Digestion relies heavily on water. It assists in breaking down nutrients, enabling your body to absorb them effectively. Inadequate hydration can lead to constipation, as the intestines need water to help move waste along. Drinking enough fluids supports a healthy gut microbiome, enhancing overall digestive health.

The skin also benefits from hydration. Water helps maintain elasticity and moisture, reducing the appearance of dryness and wrinkles. Proper hydration can improve skin tone and texture, making it look healthier. Your skin can appear lifeless when you are dehydrated. Drinking enough water is key to keeping your skin vibrant and supple.

Hydration extends beyond just drinking water. It involves understanding how much you need and how to achieve it. Factors like age, weight, activity level, and climate all influence your hydration needs. The more active you are, the more fluid you require to replace what you lose through sweat. On hot days, or during intense workouts, you may need additional fluids to stay on track.

Hydration Strategies for Optimal Health

Start with simple strategies to enhance hydration. Always have a water bottle nearby during the day. It serves as a visual cue to encourage you to drink more frequently. Aim to fill it multiple times, tracking your intake. Many people find it easier to sip regularly than to gulp down large amounts at once.

Create a routine around drinking water. Try drinking a glass first thing in the morning to kickstart your hydration. Before each meal, have another glass. This not only hydrates but can help control appetite, as thirst is sometimes mistaken for hunger.

Infusing water with fruits or herbs can enhance flavor and encourage consumption. Citrus fruits, berries, mint, or cucumber can make plain water more appealing. The added vitamins and antioxidants provide an extra health boost.

If you struggle to drink enough water, consider incorporating hydration-focused foods into your diet. Fruits and vegetables that are high in water can help you meet your daily hydration needs. Great choices include watermelon, cucumbers, oranges and strawberries. Salads loaded with greens can also help keep you hydrated while providing essential nutrients.

Set hydration goals. For many, a target of eight 8-ounce glasses of water a day works well, but individual needs vary. Pay attention to your body's signals. Other indicators include dry mouth, fatigue, or dark yellow urine. Keeping a hydration diary can help you track your intake and recognize patterns.

While water is essential, beverages like herbal teas and broths can also contribute to hydration. Unsweetened drinks, especially those without caffeine, can provide variety without excess calories. Monitor caffeine intake, as it can have a mild diuretic effect, potentially increasing fluid loss.

Alcohol can dehydrate the body. If you choose to drink, do so in moderation and balance it with water. Aim for a glass of water between alcoholic beverages to mitigate dehydration effects. This strategy not only supports hydration but also helps regulate consumption.

Sometimes, you may need to adjust your hydration strategies based on the environment. In hot weather or high altitudes, your body loses water more quickly. Be proactive about increasing fluid intake in these situations. Listen to your body. If you feel thirsty, drink. If you feel fatigued or lightheaded, you may need more water.

Athletes and those who engage in vigorous exercise should pay extra attention to hydration. Sweating significantly increases fluid needs. When you are doing your workout, consider drinking water during and after the training section. For longer sessions, electrolyte beverages can help replenish lost minerals, especially sodium and potassium. Understanding hydration is essential for maintaining health. Small changes can make a significant difference. Experiment with strategies, monitor your body's needs and stay attuned to hydrogen's role in overall well-being.

The Impact of Dehydration

Dehydration affects your body in numerous ways. Even slight dehydration can cause tiredness, lower focus, and diminished physical appearance. Your brain can become sluggish, impacting decision-making and mood. You may feel irritable or lethargic when your fluid levels drop.

Severe dehydration can lead to serious health issues. It can affect kidney function, leading to the risk of kidney stones or urinary tract infections. Chronic dehydration may contribute to constipation and digestive problems. Your body struggles to filter waste efficiently without adequate water.

Signs of dehydration can manifest in various forms. Thirst is the most common indicator, but it's not always the first sign. Look for dry mouth, fatigue, dark urine, and dizziness. In children, signs include a dry diaper for several hours or irritability.

Hydration levels can affect physical performance. If you're exercising and dehydrated, your endurance declines and recovery takes longer. Research shows that even a 2% decrease in body weight from fluid loss can impair performance. Staying hydrated helps maintain stamina and strength during workouts.

The impact of dehydration on the elderly can be particularly significant. The sense of taste diminishes as people age. This can lead to unintentional dehydration. Older adults should make a conscious effort to drink enough fluids, as they may not feel thirsty even when their bodies need water. Caregivers should encourage regular fluid intake to prevent complications.

Mental health also links closely to hydration. Studies indicate that dehydration can affect mood, increasing feelings of anxiety and stress. Adequate hydration can enhance cognitive function, potentially improving overall mental well-being. By prioritizing water intake, you support both physical and mental health

Certain medical conditions can exacerbate dehydration risks. Conditions like diabetes can increase fluid loss, requiring increased hydration efforts. Similarly, gastrointestinal illnesses may lead to fluid loss through vomiting or diarrhea. In such cases, replenishing fluids and electrolytes is crucial for recovery.

Stay proactive about hydration, especially during illness. Drink plenty of fluids to support recovery and prevent further dehydration. Monitoring symptoms and adjusting intake can help manage health effectively.

Hydrating Foods and Beverages

Many foods offer hydration benefits beyond plain water. Fruits and vegetables that contain a lot of water can help increase your fluid intake. Watermelon is about 92% water, making it an excellent choice on hot days. Cucumbers, celery, and strawberries also pack a hydrating punch.

A fruit salad with watermelon, oranges, and strawberries can refresh and nourish. Add cucumbers to salads or sandwiches for a crunchy, hydrating boost. Blending smoothies with hydrating ingredients can create a delicious way to meet your fluid needs.

Soups and broths serve as great hydration sources. Homemade vegetable soups can be packed with nutrients while contributing to overall fluid intake. Opt for low-sodium versions to minimize salt intake. Broths can also provide electrolytes, especially when recovering from illness.

Herbal teas, whether hot or cold, are another excellent option. They come in various flavors and can be enjoyed at any time of day. Opt for caffeine-free varieties, particularly if you're sensitive to caffeine's diuretic effects. Herbal teas made from ingredients like hibiscus, chamomile, or peppermint can be refreshing and hydrating.

Smoothies can be hydrating, especially when made with water-rich fruits and vegetables. Blend spinach, kale, and bananas with water or coconut water for a nutrient-packed drink. Adding chia seeds can increase fiber content and help maintain hydration.

Coconut water is a natural source of hydration and electrolyte. Its balance of sodium, potassium, and magnesium makes it an excellent post-workout beverage. It offers a light, refreshing alternative to sugary sports drinks.

When considering hydration, watch out for sugary drinks. Sodas and sweetened beverages can lead to excess calorie consumption without offering substantial hydration benefits. While they may quench thirst temporarily, they often contribute to long-term health issues.

Consider sparkling water as a flavorful alternative to soda. It offers the fizz without added sugars. You can infuse it with fruits or herbs for an added twist. Experiment with flavors to keep your hydration routine exciting.

Incorporating a variety of hydrating foods and beverages can keep hydration enjoyable.

The more variety you consume, the broader the range of nutrients and hydration benefits you receive.

Remember that hydration is a continuous process. With the right strategies, staying hydrated can become a natural part of your daily routine, promoting optimal health and well-being.

The Connection Between Nutrition and Mental Health

Diet impacts mood more than many realize. It's not just about calories; it's about how food choices shape our mental well-being. Every bite we take has the potential to influence our brain chemistry, emotional state, and overall mental health.

When you consume whole foods rich in nutrients, your body and brain benefit. Nutrients play crucial roles in neurotransmitter production. For instance, omega-3 fatty acids found in fatty fish support brain function and may reduce symptoms of depression. Foods high in antioxidants, like berries and leafy greens, combat oxidative stress and inflammation, both linked to mood disorders.

Consider the impact of carbohydrates on serotonin, the "feel-good" neurotransmitter. Complex carbohydrates, such as whole grains, can help maintain stable blood sugar levels, leading to steady energy and improved mood. Simple sugars, on the other hand, lead to spikes and crashes, contributing to irritability and mood swings.

Vitamins and minerals play an important role in mental health as well. For example, vitamin D, often gained through sunlight but also found in fortified foods, plays a vital role in mood regulation. Magnesium, found in nuts and seeds, helps with relaxation and reduces anxiety.

Some nutrients have a particularly strong connection to mood. Folate, abundant in legumes and dark greens, has been shown to combat depression. Similarly, B vitamins, found in whole grains, meat, and dairy, are essential for energy production and brain health.

While some foods enhance mental wellness, others can hinder it. Processed foods, laden with sugars and unhealthy fats, can exacerbate mood disorders. Diets high in trans fats have been linked to an increased risk of depression. Similarly, excessive consumption of caffeine can lead to anxiety and irritability.

Alcohol poses its own set of problems. While it may initially seem relaxing, it disrupts neurotransmitter balance and can lead to increased feelings of depression and anxiety over time. Being mindful of what you consume can be crucial for maintaining a balanced mood.

Mindful eating is a powerful tool. It encourages awareness of food choices and their effects on the body and mind. By slowing down and savoring each bite, you not only enjoy your meal more but also tune in to how it makes you feel. This practice can help in identifying foods that enhance or detract from your mental state. Pay attention to hunger cues. This awareness can foster healthier relationships with food. When you choose foods that nourish both body and mind, you set the stage for better mental health.

Meal planning can also enhance mindful eating. By preparing healthy meals in advance, you avoid the pitfalls of last-minute, less nutritious choices. Keep a variety of colorful fruits and vegetables on hand to ensure a nutrient-rich diet.

Listen to your body. If certain foods make you feel sluggish or irritable, it may be time to reevaluate your choices. Keeping a food diary can be a useful practice. Keep a record of your meal and your feelings afterward. This can reveal patterns and help you make informed decisions about your diet.

Incorporating regular meals and snacks helps maintain stable blood sugar levels, which in turn supports mood stability. Missing meals can cause irritability and reduce concentration. Strive for a balanced intake of macronutrients, carbohydrates, protein and fats.

Engaging in the community around food can also be beneficial. Sharing meals with friends or family fosters connection and can enhance the enjoyment of eating. This social aspect of dining can boost mood and create positive associations with food.

Experiment with new recipes that highlight whole, nutrient-dense foods. Try to make cooking a fun and creative outlet rather than a chore.

Hydration is another critical factor in mental health. Dehydration can lead to fatigue and irritability. Herbal teas can also be a soothing choice that provides hydration without caffeine.

Consider the power of herbs and spices. Turmeric, for example, has anti-inflammatory properties and may benefit mood. Similarly, omega-3-rich foods like flaxseeds and walnuts can help combat depressive symptoms. Incorporating these into your diet can provide added mental health benefits.

The gut-brain connection is another important aspect. The

gut-brain connection is crucial as the gut microbiome affects brain function and mood. Consuming a fiber-rich diet with fruits, vegetables, and whole grains a healthy gut. Probiotics found in fermented foods like yogurt and kimchi can also contribute to gut health and, consequently, mental well-being.

Avoiding food marketing traps is essential. Many processed foods are marketed as healthy but contain hidden sugars and unhealthy fats. Learning to read labels can empower you to make better choices.

A colorful plate often signifies a variety of vitamins and minerals. Explore different cuisines and seasonal produce to keep meals interesting and nutritious.

Mental health isn't just about what you eat but also how you approach food. Building a positive relationship with food involves kindness and patience. Treat yourself to your favorite meals occasionally without guilt.

Remember that mental wellness is a journey. Small, consistent changes in diet can lead to significant improvements over time. Focus on progress rather than perfection. Celebrate the positive choices you make and the way they contribute to your overall well-being.

Lastly, don't underestimate the role of physical activity. Exercise releases endorphins, which enhance mood. Combine a nutritious diet with regular physical activity for a holistic approach to mental health.

Taking charge of your nutrition can empower you to improve your mental health. Start by making small adjustments to your diet, focusing on whole, unprocessed foods. Pay attention to how these changes affect your mood and mental clarity.

By prioritizing nutrition, you pave the way for better mental health and a more balanced life.

Plant-Based Diets: Benefits and Basics

More people are discovering the advantages of eating primarily plants. Research consistently shows that plant-based nutrition can lead to lower rates of chronic diseases, better weight management, and improved overall health.

Plant-based eating focuses on whole foods, such as fruits, vegetables, whole grains, legumes, nuts, and seeds. This approach emphasizes foods in their natural state, avoiding highly processed options. A plant-based diet doesn't necessarily mean vegetarian or vegan; it simply prioritizes plant foods.

Understanding plant-based nutrition requires knowing what foods contribute to a balanced diet. Fruits and vegetables are the cornerstones. They provide essential vitamins, minerals, and fiber. Whole grains, such as brown rice and quinoa, supply energy and additional nutrients. Legumes, including beans, lentils, and chickpeas, offer protein and fiber, making them an excellent meat alternative.

Key nutrients in plant-based diets include protein, iron, calcium, omega-3 fatty acids, and vitamin B12. Contrary to common misconceptions, getting enough protein from plants is entirely possible. Legumes, nuts, seeds, and whole grains all contribute ample protein.

However, pairing iron-rich foods with vitamin C sources enhances absorption. For example, adding bell peppers to a bean salad boosts iron uptake.

Calcium is often associated with dairy, but plenty of plant foods provide this vital nutrient. Dark leafy greens, almonds, and fortified plant milks are excellent sources. Ensuring adequate calcium intake is important for bone health, especially in a plant-based diet.

These sources provide ALA, a type of omega-3 that the body can convert, albeit inefficiently, into the more active forms found in fish. Including these foods regularly supports heart and brain health.

Vitamin B12 is unique; it primarily comes from animal products. Those following a strict plant-based diet should consider fortified foods or supplements to prevent deficiency. Nutritional yeast, fortified plant milk, and cereals can be excellent sources.

Start by gradually incorporating more plant foods into meals.

Begin with a few meatless meals each week, then increase as you feel comfortable. This gradual shift makes the transition less overwhelming.

Explore new recipes and cooking methods. Try roasting vegetables, making smoothies, or experimenting with grains. Discover the vast array of flavors and textures that plant foods offer. Don't hesitate to try unfamiliar ingredients; this can lead to delightful culinary surprises.

Meal planning simplifies the transition. Set aside time each week to plan meals, ensuring a variety of nutrients. Batch cooking can save time and help maintain a plant-based focus. Prepare grains, beans, and roasted vegetables in advance for easy meal assembly.

Learn to read labels. Many packaged foods contain hidden animal products or unhealthy additives. Look for whole foods and avoid those high in sugars, unhealthy fats, and artificial ingredients.

Eating out can also be manageable. Many restaurants

offer plant-based options. Discover local eateries that specialize in plant-based cuisine. Enjoying meals in diverse settings can enhance your experience.

Stay connected with a supportive community. Engage with others interested in plant-based living, whether online or in person. Community fosters a sense of belonging and encourages healthier choices.

Delicious plant-based recipes abound. Start with simple dishes that highlight whole foods. Lunch can feature a hearty salad. Combine leafy greens, cherry tomatoes, cucumber, avocado, and chickpeas. This meal is refreshing, packed with nutrients, and satisfying.

For dinner, try a vegetable stir-fry. Sauté a variety of vibrant vegetables such as bell pepper, broccoli and snap peas in a small amount of olive oil. This dish is quick to make and loaded with nutrients.

Snacks play a vital role too. Hummus with carrot sticks or apple slices is a nutritious choice. Energy balls made from oats, nut butter, and seeds provide a quick pick-me-up. These options are simple, tasty, and easy to prepare in advance.

Desserts can also be plant-based. Experiment with banana ice cream by blending frozen bananas until creamy. This simple treat is naturally sweet and satisfying. Alternatively, bake a batch of black bean brownies for a nutritious twist on a classic dessert.

Using herbs and spices enhances flavors without adding calories. Experiment with garlic, ginger, basil, and cumin to transform simple ingredients into flavorful meals. This approach makes plant-based cooking exciting and enjoyable.

Don't forget the importance of hydration. Water is crucial for overall health. Herbal teas can add variety and provide additional health benefits. Staying hydrated supports digestion, energy levels, and mental clarity.

Navigating social situations can be challenging, but it's manageable. Offer to bring a dish to gatherings, ensuring there's something plant-based for you to enjoy. Sharing your favorite recipes can introduce others to the joys of plant-based eating.

Consider the environmental impact of your food choices. Plant-based diets generally produce less carbon emission than those rich in animal products.. Choosing local, seasonal produce can further reduce environmental impact while supporting local farmers.

Shopping for plant-based foods can be an adventure. Explore farmers' markets for fresh, seasonal produce. Look for bulk bins for grains, nuts, and seeds, which often reduce packaging waste. Familiarize yourself with local stores that carry a variety of plant-based products.

Ultimately, a plant-based diet is about making conscious choices that align with your health goals and values. Focus on the positive aspects of eating more plants. Enjoy the journey and embrace the flavors, colors, and experiences that come with it.

They contribute to broader social and environmental changes. Advocating for plant-based options in your community can inspire others to make healthier choices too.

Remember, you don't have to be perfect. Enjoy the flexibility of a plant-based lifestyle. Focus on progress, not perfection.

This way of eating can lead to vibrant health and a more fulfilling life. Explore new flavors, discover new recipes, and connect with others. Let your journey into plant-based living be a source of joy and nourishment.

The Role of Protein in Your Diet

Protein plays a crucial role in overall health. Protein is required for every cell in your body to function properly. It's crucial for tissue growth and repair, enzymes and hormone production and maintaining immune function. Without enough protein, your body can't perform these vital tasks effectively. Understanding protein's role in your diet is fundamental to maintaining good health.

Different sources of protein exist, and they fall into two main categories: animal-based and plant-based. Animal products consist of meat, poultry, fish, dairy and eggs. These foods offer complete protein, which means they provide all nine essential amino acids that the body is unable to produce. For example, chicken and salmon are excellent sources of high-quality protein, containing all necessary amino acids.

Plant-based proteins come from foods like legumes, nuts, seeds, and whole grains. While many plant proteins are considered incomplete—lacking one or more essential amino acids—they can still provide all necessary amino acids when combined properly. For example, when combined, rice and beans create complete protein. Quinoa stands out as a plant source that is complete on its own.

Exploring various protein sources can enhance your diet. Beans and lentils are rich in fiber, promoting digestive health and providing steady energy. Nuts and seeds, such as almonds and chia seeds, offer healthy fats alongside protein. Whole grains like oats and barley also contribute to your protein intake while delivering complex carbohydrates.

Quality of protein matters. Not all proteins are created equal. High-quality protein sources provide essential amino acids, while lower-quality sources may lack some. Animal proteins generally offer higher quality, but the body can thrive on high-quality plant proteins as well. It's essential to focus on a diverse range of protein sources to ensure you're meeting your nutritional needs.

Plant proteins come with additional benefits. They tend to be lower in saturated fat and cholesterol than animal proteins, promoting heart health. Consuming a variety of plant proteins can also provide a range of nutrients, such as vitamins, minerals, and antioxidants. Incorporating these into your diet can support overall wellness and reduce the risk of chronic diseases.

When choosing animal proteins, opt for lean cuts of meat and low-fat dairy. Chicken breast, fish, and beans are good choices that minimize saturated fat intake. Try to limit processed meats, which are often high in sodium and preservatives. Fresh fish, especially fatty varieties like salmon, not only provide protein but also omega-3 fatty acids beneficial for heart health.

Calculating your protein needs can help you tailor your diet. The general guideline suggests that adults require about 0.8 grams of protein per kilogram of body weight. For example, if you weigh 70 kilograms, aim for around 56 grams of protein daily. Some studies suggest that athletes would benefit from 1.2 to 2.0 grams of protein per kilogram of body weight. Consuming protein-rich foods around workouts can enhance recovery. Foods like Greek yogurt, protein smoothies, or a handful of nuts make excellent post-exercise snacks.

Older adults are also unique. As people age, muscle mass tends to decline, and adequate protein intake becomes essential for maintaining strength and functionality. Older adults should aim for higher protein intake—around 1.0 to 1.2 grams per kilogram of body weight—to support muscle health and reduce the risk of sarcopenia, the age-related loss of muscle mass.

Monitoring your protein intake can be straightforward. Keeping a food diary helps track the protein content of meals and snacks. Many mobile apps also simplify this process, allowing you to log your meals and see nutrient breakdowns. This awareness can help ensure you're meeting your protein needs throughout the day.

Combining protein-rich foods with carbohydrates and healthy fats creates balanced meals. For breakfast, try oatmeal topped with nuts and seeds for a nutritious start. Lunch might feature a quinoa salad with chickpeas and vegetables, providing a satisfying protein boost. For dinner, grilled tofu or fish alongside roasted vegetables makes for a wholesome meal.

Snacks are also an excellent opportunity to increase protein intake. Options like hummus with veggies, Greek yogurt with fruit, or a handful of mixed nuts provide both protein and essential nutrients. These snacks can help curb hunger between meals while supporting your protein goals.

Diverse cuisines offer plenty of ways to include protein in your diet. Explore recipes from various cultures that emphasize legumes, grains, and vegetables. Indian cuisine, for example, features lentils in dishes like dal, providing a delicious source of plant-based protein. Mediterranean meals often include chickpeas, which can be transformed into hummus or added to salads.

Consider food pairings to enhance protein quality. Combining grains with legumes ensures a complete amino acid profile. For instance, serving rice with black beans or lentils with whole-grain bread provides a balanced protein source. Feel free to try out various combinations to find new flavor and texture

Plant-based protein powders can be useful if you struggle to meet your protein needs through whole foods. Options like pea, hemp, or brown rice protein can supplement your diet, especially post-workout. Blending protein powder into smoothies or oatmeal can enhance nutritional value without adding significant calories.

Cooking methods influence protein quality too. Grilling, baking, and steaming help retain nutrients in proteins. Frying or heavily processing protein sources can diminish their nutritional value. Aim for cooking methods that preserve the integrity of the food while enhancing flavor.

Mindful eating practices can also support your protein goals. Are you satisfied after eating? Do certain foods give you energy or leave you sluggish? Developing a deeper connection with your food can guide you toward choices that align with your health goals.

Maintaining a balanced diet means considering other macronutrients. While protein is vital, carbohydrates and fats also play essential roles. Healthy fat from avocado, nuts and olive oil contribute to overall wellness. A balanced approach ensures you're meeting all your nutritional needs.

Protein needs vary throughout life stages. Pregnant and breastfeeding individuals require additional protein to support the growing fetus or infant. Consulting with a healthcare professional can guide protein needs during these critical periods.

Hydration is equally important when focusing on protein intake. Consuming sufficient water supplies digestion and absorption of nutrients. Staying hydrated can also help manage appetite and support overall health.

Explore plant-based protein options to diversify your diet. Tempeh, a fermented soybean product, is rich in protein and probiotics. Edamame, or young soybeans, makes for a tasty snack or addition to salads.

Seitan, made from wheat gluten, serves as a meat alternative for those seeking higher protein content.

Don't shy away from legumes. Black beans, kidney beans, and lentils are versatile and budget-friendly protein sources. They also provide fiber, which supports digestive health and keeps you feeling full.

Fermented protein sources can also benefit gut health. This can enhance digestion and nutrient absorption, including protein.

Eating a variety of foods ensures you get a broad spectrum of amino acids. Relying too heavily on one protein source can lead to imbalances. Incorporate diverse foods into your meals to maximize nutritional benefits. This approach also keeps meals interesting and flavorful.

Track changes in energy levels and physical performance as you adjust your protein intake. Increased awareness of how your body responds to different foods can help you fine-tune your diet. Adjusting your protein sources or amounts may lead to noticeable improvements in how you feel.

Consider the ethical implications of your food choices. Many people choose plant-based proteins for environmental or ethical reasons. Exploring local and sustainable protein sources can align with personal values while supporting health.

Prepare meals ahead of time to ensure you meet your protein goals. Batch cooking grains, legumes, and proteins can simplify meal prep. This practice makes it easier to assemble balanced meals quickly during busy weeks.

Enjoy the process of discovering new flavors and recipes that incorporate protein-rich foods. Engage in cooking as a creative outlet. Experimenting with spices, herbs, and cooking techniques can elevate your meals.

Protein-rich diets can enhance satiety, helping manage weight. High-protein meals can keep you feeling full longer, reducing the urge to snack on less nutritious options. This can aid in weight management while ensuring adequate nutrient intake.

Learning about different protein sources broadens your culinary horizons. Delve into international cuisines that prioritize legumes and whole grains. Explore recipes from cultures that emphasize plant-based eating, revealing new ingredients and cooking methods.

When dining out, look for menu items that highlight protein-rich ingredients. Many restaurants now offer plant-based protein options or dishes featuring legumes. Experiment with protein-enriched snacks to keep energy levels stable. Consider options like protein bars, roasted chickpeas, or edamame. These snacks can provide a convenient way to meet protein needs throughout the day.

Stay informed about the latest nutrition research. Understanding how protein impacts health can empower you to make informed choices. Research continues to reveal the benefits of protein for muscle health, weight management, and overall well-being.

Simple strategies can make a significant difference. Focus on whole, minimally processed foods that contribute to your protein intake.

As you navigate your dietary choices, remain flexible. It's okay to enjoy a variety of foods while prioritizing protein. Embrace the journey of discovering what works best for your health and lifestyle.

Fostering a positive relationship with food can enhance your overall well-being. Enjoy the flavors, textures, and experiences that come with a protein-rich diet. This approach can lead to improved health and vitality in your daily life.

Sugar: The Silent Enemy

Added sugars hide in many places. They enhance flavor, but they can harm health. Understanding what added sugars are is the first step in tackling their effects. Added sugars appear in processed foods, soft drinks, and even sauces. These sugars don't occur naturally; they're added during production. Natural sugars, on the other hand, exist in whole foods like fruits and dairy. The distinction is essential for making informed choices.

Common sources of added sugars include sweetened beverages, desserts, and snacks. This can lead to a significant excess, contributing to various health issues. Familiarizing yourself with food labels is crucial. Recognizing these ingredients empowers you to make better choices.

Health risks linked to excess sugar intake are serious. Research shows a clear connection between high sugar consumption and obesity. Not only that, but high sugar intake also correlates with an increased risk of heart disease. Studies suggest that sugar consumption raises blood pressure and promotes inflammation.

Mental health can also suffer from too much sugar. The quick energy boost from sugar may feel good initially, but it often leads to a crash. This crash can result in fatigue and irritability. Over time, high sugar intake may contribute to mood disorders.

Some studies indicate a relationship between high-sugar diets and increased rates of depression and anxiety. Balancing blood sugar levels is essential for emotional stability.

Sugar harms dental health as well. It feeds harmful bacteria in the mouth, leading to cavities and gum disease. Regular dental check-ups and proper hygiene help, but cutting back on sugar is vital for prevention.

Recognizing where sugar hides is vital for reducing consumption. Many foods labeled as healthy may still contain added sugars. Granola bars, flavored yogurts, and salad dressings can be sneaky sources. By learning to read ingredient labels, you can identify added sugars more easily.

Strategies for reducing sugar intake can make a difference. Start small. If you typically add sugar to your coffee, gradually decrease the amount. This gradual change helps your taste buds adjust over time. Focus on whole, unprocessed foods. These foods naturally contain little or no added sugars. Fresh fruits, vegetables, legumes, and whole grains provide essential nutrients without the sugar overload.

When grocery shopping, choose unsweetened products whenever possible. Look for unsweetened almond milk or yogurt. Opt for canned fruits packed in water or their juice instead of syrup. Being proactive about ingredient choices can lead to healthier eating habits.

Pay attention to portion sizes. Many snacks come in larger portions than necessary. Opt for smaller servings to enjoy treats without consuming excessive sugar. Sharing desserts can also help manage portion control while still allowing you to indulge.

Spices offer a great way to add flavor without sugar. Experiment with cinnamon, vanilla, or nutmeg in your cooking and baking. These spices enhance the taste of foods naturally, eliminating the need for added sweetness. This simple switch can transform a dish while keeping it healthy.

Healthy alternatives to sugar can satisfy your sweet cravings.

Natural sweeteners like honey and maple syrup can replace refined sugars. While they still contain sugar, they often provide additional nutrients. However, moderation is crucial, as these alternatives also affect blood sugar levels.

Consider calorie-free options such as stevia or monk fruit. These natural sweeteners provide a sweet flavor without calories. They are ideal for baking or adding to beverages. Using these substitutes can help you enjoy sweetness without the drawbacks of sugar.

The fruit serves as a fantastic alternative to processed sweets. Fresh fruit can satisfy cravings while providing vitamins, minerals, and fiber. Dried fruits are also an option, but be cautious of added sugars in some products. Blending frozen bananas creates a creamy, ice cream-like treat without added sugar.

Education about sugar content in foods empowers better decisions. Familiarize yourself with the various terms for added sugars. Learning what to look for on ingredient labels helps you navigate the supermarket more effectively. This knowledge supports healthier eating habits.

Mindful eating practices can significantly impact sugar consumption. This awareness helps you enjoy treats without overindulging. It can also lead to healthier choices as you learn to listen to your body's signals.

Making dietary changes takes time and patience. Set realistic goals for reducing sugar. Perhaps designate certain days for sugar-free meals or snacks. Gradually increase these days as you become more comfortable.

Cooking together or sharing meals can reinforce positive changes in your diet.

Incorporating more whole foods into your daily routine reduces the need for processed snacks that often contain added sugars. Fill your pantry with nuts, seeds, whole grains, and legumes. Stocking fresh produce ensures you have healthy options readily available.

When eating out, choose wisely. Many restaurants now offer healthier options. Look for dishes that focus on whole ingredients and avoid those with sugary sauces. Don't hesitate to ask for modifications to your meal to reduce sugar content.

Keeping a food diary can help you track your sugar intake. Write down what you eat, how much sugar is in those foods, and how you feel afterward. This practice raises awareness and helps you identify patterns in your consumption.

Staying hydrated is essential. Drinking plenty of water throughout the day can help manage cravings and improve overall health. Herbal teas provide variety without added sugars, making them a good alternative.

Reducing sugar doesn't mean eliminating sweetness. Finding a balance is crucial. Allow yourself occasional treats without guilt. Enjoying your favorite dessert occasionally can be part of a healthy lifestyle, as long as it's consumed in moderation.

As you reduce sugar intake, pay attention to how your body feels. Many people experience increased energy levels, better mood stability, and improved sleep. Noticing these benefits can motivate you to stick with healthier eating habits.

Creating a supportive environment at home helps maintain progress. Remove sugary snacks from your kitchen and replace them with healthier options. Stock your pantry with whole foods that align with your health goals, making better choices easier.

Explore recipes that incorporate healthy alternatives to sugar. Plenty of resources are available online, offering inspiration for meals and snacks that satisfy your sweet tooth without excessive sugar. Cooking and baking can become enjoyable activities that foster healthier habits.

Educating yourself about the broader impact of sugar consumption can strengthen your resolve. Understanding how sugar affects the body enables you to make informed choices. This knowledge can also empower you to advocate for better nutrition within your community.

Consider the long-term health benefits of reducing sugar. Lowering sugar intake can lead to weight loss, improved heart health, and a reduced risk of chronic diseases. Focusing on these advantages can motivate you to continue making healthier choices.

Patience is key as you navigate dietary changes. Adjustments take time, and it's normal to face challenges along the way. Embrace the journey and be kind to yourself as you work towards a healthier lifestyle.

As you build healthier habits, remember the importance of balance. Enjoy foods you love while incorporating more nutritious options. This approach fosters a sustainable lifestyle that supports long-term health.

Stay informed about nutrition and sugar's role in health. Engaging with new research can help you stay up-to-date on dietary guidelines and trends. This knowledge can inform your choices and promote better health.

Incorporating mindfulness into your eating practices fosters a healthier relationship with food. Practice gratitude for the nourishment that food provides, and appreciate the flavors and textures. This awareness can transform your perspective on meals and snacks.

Reducing added sugar can lead to a healthier, more vibrant life. Focus on the positive changes that accompany cutting back, and embrace the journey toward better health. Celebrate progress, stay motivated, and explore the delicious world of wholesome foods.

Fats: The Good, the Bad, and the Essential

Dietary fats often spark confusion. They play crucial roles in our bodies, yet many fear them. Understanding the different types of fats can clear up misconceptions. Fats can be divided into several categories: saturated, unsaturated, and trans fats. Each type affects health differently, making it essential to know what to include in your diet.

Saturated fats primarily come from animal sources. Foods like butter, cheese, and fatty cuts of meat contain high levels of saturated fat. While the body needs some saturated fat, excessive intake can raise cholesterol levels. This elevation in cholesterol is linked to heart disease. Recent research shows that certain sources, like coconut oil and dark chocolate, may not have the same detrimental effects when consumed in moderation.

Unsaturated fats, in contrast, are beneficial for health. These fats can help lower bad cholesterol levels, improving heart health. Polyunsaturated fats, including omega-3 and omega-6 fatty acids, come from fatty fish, flaxseeds, walnuts, and sunflower oil. Omega-3s, in particular, offer numerous health benefits, including anti-inflammatory properties and support for brain health.

Incorporating healthy fats into your diet is simple. Start by swapping out saturated fats for unsaturated ones. Adding avocado to salads or sandwiches boosts flavor and nutrition. Nuts and seeds make excellent snacks, providing a source of healthy fats and protein. These choices not only enhance your meals but also support overall health.

Understanding the importance of omega-3 fatty acids cannot be overstated. These fats play a vital role in brain function and may help reduce the risk of chronic diseases. If you're not a fish lover, consider plant-based sources such as chia seeds, flaxseeds, and walnuts. Omega-3 supplements can also provide an alternative if dietary intake is insufficient.

They are often found in margarine, shortening, and many fried and processed foods. These fats raise bad cholesterol levels while lowering good cholesterol, significantly increasing the risk of heart disease. Many countries have implemented bans on trans fats in food products. Check labels carefully, and steer clear of items containing partially hydrogenated oils.

Cooking with fats safely is essential for preserving their

health benefits. Different fats have varying smoke points—the temperature at which they start to break down and produce harmful compounds. Oils like olive oil and avocado oil have higher smoke points and are better suited for cooking at higher temperatures. On the other hand, oils like flaxseed oil are better used in salad dressings or drizzled over finished dishes. Understanding the smoke point of your cooking fats helps ensure you maximize their nutritional benefits while minimizing health risks.

Using fats in moderation is also essential. Portion control matters. Even when using olive oil or avocados, be mindful of the quantities you consume. A little can go a long way in enhancing flavor and nutrition without overloading on calories.

Incorporating a variety of fats into your diet promotes balance. Aim for diversity in your fat sources. This approach helps ensure you receive a range of nutrients and health benefits. Nuts, seeds, avocados, and olive oil provide different types of beneficial fats. Enjoying a variety of these foods can contribute to better health outcomes.

Reading labels can help you make informed choices about fats. Familiarize yourself with terms that indicate the type of fat in a product. Look for foods that list healthy fats as primary ingredients.

Avoid products with trans fats or high levels of saturated fats. Knowledge is power when it comes to making better dietary decisions.

Understanding how fats impact your body can motivate you to make healthier choices. Fats play roles in hormone production, nutrient absorption, and energy levels. They are essential for overall health. Recognizing the importance of fats can help you approach your diet more positively.

Experimenting with cooking oils can be a fun way to discover new flavors. Try different oils in dressings, marinades, or sautéing vegetables. This experimentation can make healthy eating enjoyable and exciting.

Don't forget about fat-soluble vitamins... Including healthy fats in your meals helps your body utilize these essential nutrients. Pairing colorful vegetables with healthy fats enhances nutrient absorption. For instance, drizzling olive oil over a salad can improve the absorption of vitamins from the greens.

Cooking methods also impact the quality of fats in your meals. Steaming, roasting, and sautéing with healthy oils are excellent options. Avoid frying whenever possible, as it often requires unhealthy fats. Grilling and baking are other healthier cooking methods that preserve fat quality while adding flavor.

Making conscious choices about fats can enhance your overall health. Focus on incorporating healthy fats into your daily meals. Be intentional about reducing saturated and trans fats. Simple swaps can create lasting changes.

Try new recipes that emphasize healthy fats. Explore Mediterranean dishes that feature olive oil, nuts, and fresh vegetables. Cooking with whole foods helps you appreciate the benefits of fats in a flavorful way.

Creating a balanced plate is key. Aim to include healthy fats along with proteins and carbohydrates in your meals. Consider meals that feature whole grains, lean proteins, and a variety of colorful vegetables topped with healthy fats.

Snack smartly by incorporating healthy fats. Choose nuts, seeds, or nut butter for quick, nutritious snacks. These options provide energy while offering essential nutrients. Avoid processed snacks that are often loaded with unhealthy fats and sugars.

Encouraging family and friends to embrace healthy fats can create a supportive environment. Share recipes, cooking tips, and ideas for incorporating healthy fats into meals. Cooking together can foster a sense of community while promoting better health.

Staying informed about current nutrition research can enhance your understanding of dietary fats. New studies frequently emerge, shedding light on the roles of fats in health. Engaging with reputable sources can provide clarity and guidance.

Creating meals centered around healthy fats can be a delightful culinary journey. Explore global cuisines that prioritize fats. Many cultures feature dishes rich in healthy oils, nuts, and seeds. Discovering these flavors can inspire you to make healthier choices while enjoying the variety.

Don't hesitate to seek professional advice if you have questions about dietary fats. They can help you navigate fat intake in the context of your overall diet.

Indulging in treats occasionally is okay, as long as it fits within a balanced approach. Focus on enjoying meals while being mindful of fat sources.

Reflecting on your dietary choices can be a powerful tool. Pay attention to energy levels, mood, and overall health. This awareness can guide you toward making better choices in the future.

Simple recipes that highlight these fats can be quick and satisfying. Tossing vegetables in olive oil and roasting them is an easy way to incorporate healthy fats into your meals.

Consider the broader impact of your dietary choices. Emphasizing healthy fats supports not only personal health but also sustainability. Many plant-based fats come from sources that are better for the environment. Making mindful choices can contribute to a healthier planet.

Recognizing the essential roles of fats can shift your perspective. Rather than fearing fats, embrace them as vital components of a nutritious diet.

Experimenting with fat-based sauces and dressings can enhance meals. Homemade dressings using olive oil, vinegar, and herbs are flavorful and nutritious. These alternatives allow you to control the ingredients while adding delicious flavors to your dishes.

Remember that health is a journey. Embracing healthy fats as part of your diet can enhance well-being and vitality. Focus on making choices that align with your health goals, and enjoy the process of discovery along the way.

Meal Planning for Optimal Health

Meal planning brings structure to eating. It can transform chaotic food choices into thoughtful decisions. The benefits are numerous. When you plan meals, you save time, reduce stress, and often eat healthier. Knowing what to eat ahead of time helps prevent impulsive decisions that lead to unhealthy choices. You gain control over your diet and make it easier to incorporate nutritious foods.

Meal planning saves money too. When you buy ingredients with specific meals in mind, you avoid unnecessary purchases. This approach minimizes food waste and helps you stick to your budget. Plus, cooking at home generally costs less than dining out. Planning allows you to make the most of your grocery budget while ensuring you have healthy options at hand.

Creating balanced meals is essential for optimal health.

Ensure that each meal offers a balanced mix of macronutrients. For example, a plate might consist of half of vegetables, a quarter of whole grains, and a quarter of protein.

Start by choosing a protein source for your meals. For plant-based options, consider tofu, tempeh, or quinoa. Next, include plenty of vegetables. Colorful vegetables not only add nutrients but also make your plate visually appealing. Aim for a variety of colors; this ensures a range of vitamins and minerals.

Whole grains should play a significant role in your meals. Options like brown rice, quinoa, farro, and whole-grain pasta offer fiber and energy. Incorporating these grains supports digestive health and provides lasting energy throughout the day. Finally, add healthy fats to your meals. Nuts, seeds, avocado, and olive oil contribute flavor and essential fatty acids.

The process of creating balanced meals begins with planning. Start with a weekly menu. Each meal should follow the balance of proteins, grains, vegetables, and fats. Flexibility is key, so adjust meals based on what's in season or on sale.

Quick and easy meal prep ideas make planning less overwhelming. Cook a big batch of quinoa or brown rice that you can use throughout the week. Prepping proteins in advance helps too. Grill chicken breasts or bake salmon for quick meals later.

Make use of simple recipes that require minimal effort. One-pot dishes, sheet pan meals, or slow cooker recipes can save time and clean up. Consider making a large vegetable stir-fry, where you can toss in whatever veggies you have on hand, along with tofu or chicken, and serve it over rice. This method is not only efficient but also allows for creativity with flavors and ingredients.

Batch cooking is another effective strategy. Prepare larger quantities of meals to freeze for later. Soups, stews, and casseroles freeze well. When you batch cook, you create easy options for busy days. Label containers with dates and contents for easy identification later. This strategy ensures you have healthy meals on hand, preventing the temptation of takeout.

Smoothies are another quick meal option. Blend fruits, leafy greens, and a protein source like yogurt or nut butter for a nutritious breakfast or snack. Prepare smoothie packs by portioning out ingredients in bags and freezing them. This approach makes it easy to grab a healthy option on the go.

Keep your goals visible. This simple action serves as a reminder of what you want to achieve. Setting specific, measurable goals can provide clarity. For instance, aim to eat at least five servings of fruits and vegetables each day.

Mindful Eating for Better Health

It's about being present and fully engaged during meals, recognizing hunger cues, and savoring each bite. Instead of eating on autopilot, you pay attention to the colors, textures, and flavors. This approach fosters a deeper connection with what you eat and can lead to healthier choices.

What is Mindful Eating?

It asks you to notice the food's appearance, aroma, and taste. This practice shifts your attention away from distractions—like screens or multitasking—allowing you to engage fully with the meal. Mindful eating emphasizes understanding your body's signals and distinguishing between hunger and cravings.

Instead of reacting automatically to hunger, you pause to ask yourself what your body truly needs. This involves listening to your body's cues. Mindful eating empowers you to make conscious decisions rather than reacting impulsively.

The origins of mindful eating can be traced back to Buddhist teachings, where mindfulness itself is a core principle. It teaches awareness, encouraging individuals to cultivate a more thoughtful relationship with their food. This doesn't mean strict rules; rather, it invites you to explore your habits, making adjustments as needed.

Techniques for Practicing Mindfulness

Implementing mindfulness in your eating habits doesn't require a drastic overhaul of your lifestyle. Start with simple techniques that gradually build your awareness.

1. Create a Calm Environment

Start by setting the scene. Turn off the TV, silence your phone, and sit at a table instead of eating on the couch. A peaceful environment allows you to focus entirely on your meal.

2. Engage Your Senses

Before you take a bite, observe your food. Look at the colors and shapes. Smell the aromas. Notice the temperature and texture. Engaging your senses heightens your awareness and enriches the eating experience.

3. Take Smaller Bites

Instead of cramming food into your mouth, take smaller bites. This simple change forces you to chew more thoroughly, enhancing your appreciation of the flavors and textures. It also slows down the eating process, allowing your brain time to register fullness.

4. Chew Thoroughly

Chewing is crucial. This not only aids digestion but also extends the eating experience. Each chew reveals new flavors, making each bite more satisfying.

5. Pause Between Bites

After each bite, put down your utensils. Are you still hungry? This pause encourages reflection and helps you recognize when you're satisfied.

6. Reflect on Your Food

Consider where your food comes from. Think about the farmers, the land, and the processes involved in bringing it to your plate. This connection can deepen your appreciation and lead to more conscious choices.

7. Practice Gratitude

Before eating, take a moment to express gratitude. Acknowledge the effort involved in creating your meal. This practice fosters a positive mindset and reinforces a healthy relationship with food.

8. Notice Your Thoughts and Feelings

As you eat, thoughts and feelings may arise. Acknowledge them without judgment. If you feel anxious or guilty, notice these emotions and gently refocus on your meal. This awareness can help you develop a more compassionate relationship with yourself and your food.

9. Use Mindful Eating Apps

Consider using apps designed to promote mindfulness in eating. Many offer guided exercises and reminders to pause and reflect. These tools can support your journey towards more mindful eating habits.

10. Make It a Social Activity

Invite friends or family to join you in a mindful eating experience. Discuss your meals, share your thoughts, and encourage one another to engage fully. This social aspect can enhance the enjoyment of food and reinforce mindful practices.

The Benefits of Slowing Down

The benefits of mindful eating extend far beyond immediate enjoyment. Slowing down has a profound impact on both physical and mental health.

1. Improved Digestion

Eating slowly aids digestion. Chewing food thoroughly breaks it down, allowing enzymes to do their job more effectively.

2. Better Portion Control guy

When you eat mindfully, you become more attuned to your body's hunger signals. This awareness helps prevent overeating. You learn to recognize when you're satisfied rather than continuing to eat out of habit.

3. Enhanced Satisfaction

Mindful eating fosters a deeper appreciation of food. By savoring flavors and textures, meals become more enjoyable. This heightened satisfaction can reduce the desire for unhealthy snacks later.

4. Weight Management

Many studies suggest that mindful eating supports weight loss and management. By promoting awareness and reducing emotional eating, this practice helps individuals make healthier choices and maintain a balanced diet.

5. Emotional Balance

Mindful eating can help address emotional eating. By tuning into your feelings before reaching for food, you can distinguish between genuine hunger and emotional cravings. This awareness fosters healthier coping mechanisms.

6. Increased Awareness of Food Choices

Mindful eating encourages conscious decision-making. You become more aware of the nutritional value of your food, leading to better choices. This heightened awareness promotes a diet rich in fruits, vegetables, whole grains, and lean proteins.

7. Stress Reduction

Practicing mindfulness in any form can reduce stress. Eating mindfully slows down your pace of life, allowing you to relax and enjoy the moment. This calming effect can carry over into other areas of your life.

8. Strengthened Relationship with Food

Rather than viewing it as a source of guilt or anxiety, you begin to appreciate its role in nourishment and enjoyment.

9. Greater Connection to Body Cues

Listening to your body's hunger and fullness cues becomes second nature. You learn to trust your instincts, making food choices based on genuine needs rather than external pressures.

10. Promotion of Healthy Habits

Incorporating mindful eating into your life can inspire other healthy habits. As you become more conscious about what you eat, you may feel motivated to exercise, sleep better, and prioritize overall wellness.

Building a Healthy Relationship with Food

This approach shifts the focus from restriction and guilt to enjoyment and nourishment.

1. Let Go of Food Guilt

Many people struggle with guilt surrounding food choices. Mindful eating encourages you to release this guilt. Every food can fit into a healthy diet; the key lies in balance and moderation.

2. Redefine Healthy Eating

Instead of adhering to strict diets, redefine what healthy eating means to you. This flexibility leads to a sustainable approach.

3. Cultivate Intuition

Trusting your instincts around food is crucial. This intuitive approach fosters a sense of empowerment in your food choices.

4. Embrace Diversity in Diet

Explore different foods and cuisines. Mindful eating invites you to appreciate diversity in your meals. Experimenting with new ingredients can enhance your palate and make eating more enjoyable.

5. Prioritize Nourishment Over Restrictions

Prioritizing nourishment means filling your plate with a variety of whole, unprocessed foods that fuel your body.

6. Practice Self-Compassion

When cravings or overeating occur, practice self-compassion. Recognize that everyone has moments of indulgence. Approach these instances with kindness rather than criticism.

7. Celebrate Food as a Social Experience

Celebrate meals with friends and family, enjoying the connections and conversations that come with them. This social aspect reinforces the positive experience of eating.

8. Keep a Food Journal

Consider maintaining a food journal to reflect on your eating habits. Jot down thoughts and feelings before and after meals.

9. Develop Healthy Cooking Skills

Enhance your relationship with food by learning to cook. Cooking can be a creative outlet, allowing you to explore flavors and ingredients.

10. Be Open to Change

Stay open to change and growth. Embrace new ideas and practices that support your journey towards mindful eating.

Through mindful eating, you discover a world of flavors and

experiences. By focusing on the present moment, you foster a healthier relationship with food and enhance your overall well-being.

Nutrition Across the Lifespan

Understanding nutrition means recognizing that our needs shift as we move through different stages of life. Each phase—childhood, adolescence, adulthood, and old age—demands specific nutrients and dietary considerations. By tailoring our diets to these needs, we can support overall health and well-being.

Nutritional Needs for Different Life Stages

Infancy marks a period of rapid growth. During this stage, babies require a diet rich in essential nutrients. Breast milk or fortified formula provides the foundation, offering the perfect balance of fats, proteins, and carbohydrates. Breastfeeding offers antibodies and promotes healthy gut flora, laying the groundwork for a strong immune system.

As children grow, their nutritional needs evolve. They require adequate energy for physical activity and mental development. Key nutrients include iron, calcium, and vitamins A and D. Iron supports cognitive function and prevents anemia, while calcium is vital for bone health. Ensuring children consume a variety of fruits, vegetables, whole grains, and protein sources sets them on a path to healthy growth.

In adolescence, the body undergoes significant changes. Teens experience growth spurts and hormonal changes that increase their nutritional needs. A focus on nutrient-dense foods becomes essential. Increased protein supports muscle development, while calcium and vitamin D promote bone density. Regular meals and healthy snacks help sustain energy levels, aiding concentration during this demanding period.

Adulthood brings about a need for balanced nutrition. Individuals must focus on maintaining a healthy weight and preventing chronic diseases. A diet rich in whole foods—fruits, vegetables, whole grains, lean proteins—supports heart health and reduces the risk of conditions like diabetes and hypertension. Monitoring portion sizes becomes crucial as metabolism may slow down.

As we transition into older adulthood, nutritional needs shift again. Aging bodies require fewer calories but more nutrient-dense foods. Protein intake remains important for maintaining muscle mass. Adequate fiber supports digestive health, while hydration is crucial, as older adults may have a reduced thirst sensation. Attention to vitamins and minerals, particularly B12 and D, helps combat deficiencies common in older age.

Pregnancy and Nutrition

Pregnancy transforms a woman's body, making nutrition even more critical. The dietary choices made during this time impact both the mother's health and the developing baby. Key nutrients take center stage: folic acid, iron, calcium, and omega-3 fatty acids.

Folic acid is non-negotiable. It prevents neural tube defects and supports the healthy development of the baby's brain and spine. Women should begin supplementation before conception and continue throughout pregnancy.

Iron is vital as blood volume increases during pregnancy. The body needs iron to produce hemoglobin, which carries oxygen to brain development. Fatty fish like salmon and walnuts are excellent for both mother and baby. Consuming iron-rich foods like lean meats, beans, and spinach is essential. Pairing these with vitamin C sources—like citrus fruits—enhances absorption.

Calcium aids in the growth of the baby's bones and teeth. Dairy products, fortified plant milks, and leafy greens provide ample calcium. Adequate intake helps prevent the mother from losing her bone density.

Omega-3 fatty acids, especially DHA, play a crucial role in

sources. If seafood is limited, consider plant-based sources and supplements after consulting a healthcare provider.

Hydration also plays a key role. Pregnant women should aim to drink plenty of fluids to support increased blood volume and amniotic fluid production. Water, herbal teas, and nutrient-rich smoothies can help maintain hydration.

Additionally, mindful eating becomes essential during pregnancy. Avoiding processed foods and focusing on whole, nutrient-dense options supports both maternal health and fetal development. Women should listen to their bodies, eating when hungry and stopping when full.

Healthy Aging and Dietary Considerations

Healthy aging hinges on diet and lifestyle choices. As individuals age, maintaining physical and cognitive health becomes paramount. Nutrition plays a pivotal role in this journey, promoting longevity and quality of life.

Older adults often face challenges such as reduced appetite and changes in taste. Focusing on nutrient-dense foods becomes crucial. Choosing fruits, vegetables, whole grains, lean proteins, and healthy fats ensures that meals remain satisfying while providing essential nutrients.

Protein intake deserves special attention. It aids in preserving muscle mass, which tends to decrease as we age. Incorporating sources like beans, legumes, nuts, seeds, dairy, and lean meats can help meet protein needs. This is especially important for preventing sarcopenia, the loss of muscle mass and strength that occurs with aging.

Fiber intake is equally vital. It aids digestion and helps prevent constipation, a common issue among older adults. Staying hydrated also supports digestive health.

Vitamins and minerals become more important as the body ages.

Vitamin B12 absorption may decline, so older adults should consider fortified foods or supplements. Vitamin D supports bone health, and many older individuals may benefit from increased intake. Sunlight exposure, fortified foods, and supplements can help achieve adequate levels.

Moreover, cognitive health is a growing concern. Antioxidant-rich foods—like berries, nuts, and dark leafy greens—may help protect against cognitive decline. Omega-3 fatty acids, found in fatty fish and flaxseeds, also support brain health.

Social aspects of eating should not be overlooked. Sharing meals with family and friends can combat loneliness and enhance enjoyment. Cooking together can promote healthy eating habits and foster connections.

Physical activity complements good nutrition. Combining a nutritious diet with an active lifestyle leads to a holistic approach to healthy aging.

Special Considerations for Children

Children represent a unique group with specific nutritional needs. Their growth and development hinge on adequate nutrition, making it vital to provide a balanced diet from an early age.

Breastfeeding provides essential nutrients during infancy. It establishes healthy eating patterns and can reduce the risk of allergies and obesity later in life. When transitioning to solids, introducing a variety of foods helps children develop preferences for healthy options.

Key nutrients for young children include iron and calcium. Iron supports cognitive development, while calcium is crucial for growing bones. Incorporating foods like fortified cereals, dairy products, and green vegetables can help meet these needs.

Picky eating often surfaces during childhood. This is a normal phase, but parents can encourage healthy habits by offering a variety of foods. Repeated exposure to different flavors can help children accept new foods over time. Making meals fun—using colorful fruits and vegetables, for example—can spark interest.

Snack choices also impact nutrition. Healthy snacks—like fruit, yogurt, or nuts—fuel energy and support concentration. Avoiding sugary snacks helps prevent energy crashes and promotes better overall health.

A nutritious breakfast enhances focus and learning. Whole grains, fruits, and protein sources provide the energy needed for a productive morning.

Sitting together at the table fosters communication and encourages children to try new foods. Parents can model healthy choices, demonstrating that nutritious foods can be both delicious and satisfying.

Hydration is important for children, too. Encouraging water consumption instead of sugary drinks helps maintain energy levels and supports overall health. Involving children in choosing their beverages can empower them to make better choices.

Physical activity complements good nutrition for children. Encouraging play and exercise helps maintain a healthy weight and fosters a love for movement. Outdoor activities, sports, and active play promote both physical health and social skills. nutrition education should start early. Teaching children about food, where it comes from, and the benefits of healthy choices sets the stage for lifelong habits. Cooking together can be a fun way to impart knowledge while enjoying quality time.

By addressing the unique nutritional needs at each life stage, we can empower individuals to make informed choices. Adapting our diets to support growth, health, and longevity is a journey that begins at birth and continues throughout life. Embracing the power of nutrition ensures a better quality of life, no matter the age.

Overcoming Dietary Challenges

Navigating the landscape of healthy eating presents challenges that many people face. From financial constraints to social pressures, a variety of obstacles can hinder the journey to a nutritious diet.

Common Barriers to Healthy Eating

Time constraints often top the list of barriers. Busy schedules can make meal planning and preparation feel daunting. Fast food and convenience options frequently win out over wholesome meals. This convenience comes at a cost, both nutritionally and financially. Rushed eating can lead to poor choices, relying on processed foods that lack essential nutrients.

Lack of knowledge plays a significant role as well. Many people feel overwhelmed by conflicting information about diets, nutrition, and healthy eating. Misleading marketing can promote unhealthy foods as "healthy" alternatives, complicating decision-making. Understanding food labels and ingredients becomes crucial to discern what is truly beneficial.

Access to fresh and nutritious food can also present a challenge. Food deserts—areas with limited access to grocery stores—make it difficult to find healthy options. Convenience stores may stock processed snacks and sugary drinks, leaving little room for fresh produce. Transportation issues can exacerbate this problem, particularly for those relying on public transit or walking.

Emotional factors influence eating habits significantly. Recognizing emotional triggers is key to making more mindful choices. Social influences pose additional challenges. Family dynamics, peer pressure, and cultural traditions often dictate food choices. When others around you prioritize unhealthy options, it becomes easy to fall into similar patterns. Navigating these social pressures requires awareness and assertiveness.

Financial constraints also hinder healthy eating. Many people perceive healthy foods as expensive, leading to a preference for cheaper, processed options. In reality, eating well on a budget is possible with planning and resourcefulness. Understanding how to make cost-effective choices is essential.

Strategies for Eating Well on a Budget

Eating healthy doesn't have to break the bank. Several strategies can help you maintain a nutritious diet without overspending.

1. Plan Your Meals

Start by planning meals for the week. Make a shopping list based on the meals you plan to cook. Planning can help you avoid impulse buys and minimize food waste. Stick to your list while shopping to keep expenses in check.

2. Buy in Bulk

Buying non-perishables. Store these items properly to extend their shelf life and maximize your investment.

3. Embrace Seasonal Produce

Shopping for seasonal fruits and vegetables often saves money while ensuring freshness. Seasonal produce tends to be cheaper and tastier. Visit local farmers' markets or grocery stores that highlight seasonal items for the best deals.

4. Prioritize Whole Foods

Whole foods generally provide more nutrients and flavor for your dollar. Processed foods may appear cheaper but often lack nutritional value and lead to increased health costs over time.

5. Cook at Home

Preparing meals from scratch can be enjoyable and rewarding. Involve family members or friends to make it a fun activity, fostering healthy habits together.

6. Use Leftovers Wisely

Transform leftovers into new meals. Get creative with ingredients to minimize waste. For example, leftover roasted vegetables can become a tasty soup or stir-fry. This practice not only saves money but also reduces the environmental impact of food waste.

7. Grow Your Food

Consider starting a small garden, even if it's just herbs on a windowsill. Growing your fruits and vegetables can be both cost-effective and fulfilling. Many herbs and vegetables are easy to cultivate and require minimal space.

8. Take Advantage of Sales and Coupons

Many grocery stores offer loyalty programs that can help reduce costs. Stock up on pantry staples when they're on sale, ensuring you have nutritious options readily available.

9. Choose Plant-Based Proteins

Incorporating these into your diet not only saves money but also provides essential nutrients. Aim to create a balanced plate with a variety of proteins, grains, and vegetables.

Overcoming Dietary Challenges

Navigating the landscape of healthy eating presents challenges that many people face. From financial constraints to social pressures, a variety of obstacles can hinder the journey to a nutritious diet.

Common Barriers to Healthy Eating

Time constraints often top the list of barriers. Busy schedules can make meal planning and preparation feel daunting. Fast food and convenience options frequently win out over wholesome meals. This convenience comes at a cost, both nutritionally and financially. Rushed eating can lead to poor choices, relying on processed foods that lack essential nutrients.

Lack of knowledge plays a significant role as well. Many people feel overwhelmed by conflicting information about diets, nutrition, and healthy eating. Misleading marketing can promote unhealthy foods as "healthy" alternatives, complicating decision-making. Understanding food labels and ingredients becomes crucial to discern what is truly beneficial.

Access to fresh and nutritious food can also present a

challenge. Food deserts—areas with limited access to grocery stores—make it difficult to find healthy options. Convenience stores may stock processed snacks and sugary drinks, leaving little room for fresh produce. Transportation issues can exacerbate this problem, particularly for those relying on public transit or walking.

Emotional factors influence eating habits significantly. Recognizing emotional triggers is key to making more mindful choices. Social influences pose additional challenges. Family dynamics, peer pressure, and cultural traditions often dictate food choices. When others around you prioritize unhealthy options, it becomes easy to fall into similar patterns. Navigating these social pressures requires awareness and assertiveness.

Financial constraints also hinder healthy eating. Many people perceive healthy foods as expensive, leading to a preference for cheaper, processed options. In reality, eating well on a budget is possible with planning and resourcefulness.

Understanding how to make cost-effective choices is essential.

Dealing with Food Allergies and Intolerances

Food allergies and intolerances complicate the journey to healthy eating. Understanding how to manage these conditions is crucial for maintaining health and enjoying food.

1. Know Your Triggers

Identify specific foods that cause allergic reactions or intolerances. This may require consulting a healthcare professional for testing and diagnosis. Once you know your triggers, you can avoid them and make informed choices.

2. Read Labels Carefully

Become an expert at reading food labels. Look for hidden ingredients that may contain allergens. Manufacturers often change formulations, so it's vital to check labels each time you purchase a product.

3. Communicate Your Needs

When eating out or at social events, make sure to share your dietary restrictions. Feel free to inquire about ingredients or how dishes are prepared. Most establishments are willing to accommodate dietary needs when informed.

4. Explore Alternatives

There are numerous alternatives available for common allergens. For example, almond milk can replace dairy milk, and gluten-free grains can substitute for wheat.

5. Meal Prep

Batch-cook meals that fit your dietary needs. This approach not only saves time but also ensures you have safe options readily available.

6. Educate Friends and Family

Share your dietary needs with friends and family. Educating them about your allergies or intolerances helps create a supportive environment. They may even join you in exploring new recipes and alternatives.

7. Join Support Groups

Think about participating in support groups, whether online or in person. Engaging with others who are experiencing similar challenges can offer helpful resources and emotional support. Sharing experiences can lead to discovering new recipes and coping strategies.

8. Keep Snacks Handy

Always have safe snacks on hand. This helps avoid situations where you might feel tempted to eat something that could trigger an allergic reaction. Healthy snacks can include fruits, nuts, or homemade treats.

9. Stay Informed

Research new products and trends related to your food allergies or intolerances. The market continues to evolve, with more options becoming available. Staying informed can help you discover safe foods that fit your lifestyle.

10. Consult a Nutritionist

If managing food allergies or intolerances becomes overwhelming, consider seeking guidance from a registered dietitian or nutritionist. They can help create a balanced meal plan tailored to your needs while ensuring you receive all necessary nutrients.

Navigating Social Situations

Social events often present challenges to maintaining healthy eating habits. Food plays a significant role in gatherings, making it essential to navigate these situations mindfully.

1. Assess the Situation Ahead of Time

Before attending an event, assess what food options may be available. If possible, check the menu in advance or ask the host about what will be served. This knowledge helps you plan and prepares you for making healthy choices.

2. Eat a Healthy Snack Beforehand

Arriving at an event with a healthy snack can curb hunger and reduce the likelihood of making impulsive choices. A small serving of fruit, yogurt, or nuts can help you feel satisfied, allowing you to make mindful decisions later.

3. Bring a Dish to Share

Contribute a healthy dish to social gatherings. This ensures there's at least one nutritious option available and provides an opportunity to share healthy recipes with others. Get creative and introduce friends to delicious, wholesome foods.

4. Practice Portion Control

When faced with a buffet or multiple food options, practice portion control. Choose smaller servings of various items to satisfy cravings without overindulging. This approach allows you to enjoy a variety of flavors without compromising your health goals.

5. Focus on Enjoying the Company

Shift the focus from food to the social experience. Engage in conversations and connect with others. By prioritizing social interaction over food, you may find yourself less tempted to overeat.

6. Set Boundaries

Establish personal boundaries regarding food choices. It's okay to politely decline items that don't align with your health goals. Communicating your preferences can help you stay on track without offending others.

7. Be Mindful of Alcohol Consumption

Alcohol can contribute empty calories and impact decision-making regarding food choices. Alternating alcoholic drinks with water can help manage consumption while keeping you hydrated.

8. Find Support in Friends

Identify friends or family members who share similar dietary goals. Support from others can make social situations less daunting. Together, you can navigate food choices and motivate each other to stick to healthy habits.

9. Practice Mindfulness

When eating at social gatherings, practice mindfulness. Slowing down enhances the enjoyment of food and helps prevent overeating.

10. Don't Be Too Hard on Yourself

Remember that it's okay to indulge occasionally. Perfection isn't the goal; balance is key. Enjoying a treat in moderation won't derail your overall progress. The focus should be on long-term habits rather than individual moments.

By addressing common barriers and employing practical strategies, healthy eating becomes more achievable. Understanding individual needs and adapting to various circumstances empowers everyone to overcome dietary challenges and embrace a more nutritious lifestyle.

Building a Sustainable Eating Habit

Developing sustainable eating habits requires understanding the psychology behind habits and finding ways to make lasting changes. Habits form through repetition and reinforcement, creating patterns that become automatic over time. By focusing on these principles, you can create a healthier relationship with food.

The Psychology of Habit Formation

Habits form as the brain creates pathways in response to repeated behaviors. This process starts with a cue, followed by a routine, and ultimately leads to a reward. Recognizing these elements in your eating habits is essential for change.

Identify your cues. Do you reach for snacks when you're bored or stressed? Instead of turning to unhealthy options, consider substituting with healthier snacks like fruits or vegetables. Over time, your brain will begin to associate these healthier choices with the same cues.

The routine phase involves making choices that align with your nutritional goals. For example, if you want to increase your vegetable intake, begin by incorporating one extra serving into your meals each day. This small change can gradually build into a habit. Consistency is vital here; try to repeat this behavior daily, allowing it to become part of your routine.

The reward reinforces the habit. When you choose a healthy option, notice how it makes you feel. Maybe you have more energy or experience less bloating. Acknowledge these positive outcomes. The brain craves rewards, and highlighting the benefits of your choices strengthens the connection, making it more likely you'll continue the behavior.

Sometimes, habits become entrenched in negative thought patterns. Shifting your mindset can facilitate change. Instead of thinking, "I can't eat that," reframe it to, "I choose not to eat that." This perspective empowers you and aligns your choices with your goals. Emphasizing what you can have, rather than what you can't, creates a more positive relationship with food.

Creating small, achievable goals is crucial. Start with one change at a time. Perhaps commit to drinking an extra glass of water daily or adding a piece of fruit to breakfast. As these behaviors become habitual, build on them. Gradual changes lead to lasting results.

Setting Realistic Nutrition Goals

Setting realistic nutrition goals is vital for long-term success. Aim for clarity and specificity in your goals. Do you want to incorporate more whole foods, increase your vegetable intake, or reduce processed foods?

For instance, instead of saying, "I want to eat more vegetables," try, "I will eat at least two servings of vegetables with dinner five days a week."

Accountability plays a significant role in goal achievement. Share your objectives with friends or family. Additionally, consider joining a group or community that shares similar goals. Engaging with others provides support and inspiration.

Avoid setting overly ambitious goals. While it's great to aspire to significant changes, focusing on small, attainable steps fosters a sense of accomplishment. Each small victory builds momentum, making it easier to tackle larger goals.

Reflect regularly on your progress. Schedule time each week to assess what worked and what didn't. This practice allows for adjustments and helps maintain focus. If a particular strategy isn't effective, don't hesitate to modify it. Flexibility is essential; what works for one person may not work for another. Visual reminders can bolster your goal-setting efforts. Seeing your goals in writing serves as a constant reminder of what you're working toward. This technique reinforces commitment and can reignite motivation when it wanes.

Tracking Progress and Staying Motivated

Monitoring your progress is key to building sustainable habits. Tracking helps you recognize patterns, identify areas for improvement, and celebrate achievements. Choose a method that resonates with you, whether it's a journal, an app, or a simple spreadsheet.

Daily or weekly food logs provide insights into what you eat and when. Recording meals allows you to spot trends, such as whether you're more likely to indulge in snacks during specific times.

Use your tracking method to assess not just what you eat, but how you feel. Note your energy levels, mood, and digestion. Understanding how different foods affect your body empowers you to make better choices. For example, if you notice that a heavy meal leaves you sluggish, consider opting for lighter options next time.

Accountability partners can enhance motivation. Check in regularly to discuss progress, share tips, and encourage each other. This support system can help keep you focused and committed, especially during challenging times.

Consider setting up rewards for reaching milestones. This doesn't have to involve food; instead, think of experiences or items that excite you. Treat yourself to a movie night, a new book, or a day out once you achieve specific goals.

Stay adaptable. Life is unpredictable, and sometimes habits slip. Instead, reflect on the situation, identify triggers, and move forward. Building resilience is essential.

Utilize technology to assist your journey. Numerous apps offer meal tracking, recipes, and even communities for support. Explore options that align with your preferences and habits. Some apps can analyze your dietary intake, offering personalized feedback and suggestions for improvement.

Visual aids can enhance motivation. Create charts to visualize your progress, or set up a calendar to mark achievements. Seeing tangible proof of your efforts can be a powerful motivator.

Creating a Supportive Environment

Your environment significantly influences your eating habits. Transforming your space can facilitate healthier choices. Start by decluttering your kitchen. If you have fresh fruits and vegetables readily available, you're more likely to reach for them.

Keep healthy snacks at eye level in the pantry and fridge. When you open these spaces, your eyes naturally gravitate toward what's most visible. If you place whole foods in prominent positions, you'll find it easier to make healthier selections.

Meal prepping helps create a supportive environment. When hunger strikes, you'll have ready-to-eat, nutritious options at your fingertips. This reduces the temptation to grab processed or unhealthy foods.

Involve family or roommates in the process. Share your goals and invite them to participate in creating a healthier home environment. Cooking together, trying new recipes, or even attending local farmers' markets can turn healthy eating into a fun, shared experience. Support from loved ones can significantly boost motivation.

Modify your dining space as well. If you often eat in front of the TV, consider shifting to the dining table. This small change encourages mindful eating, allowing you to focus on your meals rather than distractions. Mindfulness enhances enjoyment and helps you tune into hunger cues.

Set boundaries around social eating situations. If you know you'll be attending a gathering with unhealthy options, plan. Eat a healthy snack before arriving to reduce the temptation to overindulge. You might also consider bringing a nutritious dish to share, ensuring you have at least one option that aligns with your goals.

Create a food-friendly social network. Engage with communities, whether online or locally, that prioritize nutrition and wellness. This environment fosters accountability and encourages shared learning.

Foster a positive mindset around food. Avoid labeling foods as "good" or "bad." This dichotomy can lead to guilt or shame when indulging in certain treats. Instead, focus on moderation and balance. Allow yourself the occasional indulgence without feeling guilty, and reinforce the idea that healthy eating is about overall patterns, not perfection.

By understanding the psychology of habit formation, setting realistic goals, tracking progress, and creating a supportive environment, you can build sustainable eating habits. Embrace the journey.

Conclusion

Recapping key nutritional strategies illuminates the path to better health. Focus on whole, plant-based foods. These foods offer essential nutrients while minimizing empty calories. Aim for variety; each color in your meal signifies different nutrients. This approach not only enhances your diet but also keeps meals exciting.

Understand the importance of fiber. It aids digestion and supports gut health. Incorporating beans, lentils, and whole grains boosts fiber intake. It helps regulate blood sugar and keeps you feeling full longer. Don't forget about healthy fats. Avocados, nuts, and seeds provide necessary nutrients while promoting heart health. Omega-3 fatty acids from flaxseeds and chia seeds are especially beneficial.

Stay hydrated. Water fuels every bodily function. Drinking

adequate amounts supports energy levels, aids digestion, and improves skin health. This small change reminds you to drink water throughout the day.

Pay attention to portion sizes. Use smaller dishes to help control portions. Mindful eating plays a crucial role here. This practice helps prevent overeating and enhances enjoyment.

Embrace meal planning. Dedicate time each week to outline your meals. This strategy not only saves time but also reduces the temptation to reach for unhealthy options. Prepare ingredients in advance. Chop vegetables or cook grains ahead of time to streamline the cooking process during the week.

Your journey to enhanced health and longevity begins with these principles. Each choice contributes to your overall well-being. Embrace the idea that small changes lead to significant impacts. Prioritize consistency over perfection

Stay curious and encourage continued learning. Nutrition science evolves, and staying informed allows you to adapt your choices. Read books, attend workshops, or follow credible health resources.

Your path forward involves embracing a healthier lifestyle. Remember, the journey isn't just about food; it encompasses physical activity, mental well-being, and overall lifestyle choices.

As you navigate this journey, embrace the joy of cooking and experimenting with new foods. Discover new flavors, try unfamiliar ingredients, and explore diverse cuisines. This mindset shift fosters a positive relationship with food and enhances your experience.

Sustainability also matters. Opt for seasonal produce, reduce waste, and support local farmers when possible. Every small action contributes to a larger goal of living healthily and responsibly.

This is your time to thrive. Embrace the challenge of building a healthier lifestyle. Stay committed, be patient with yourself, and remember that progress, not perfection, defines success.

www.ingramcontent.com/pod-product-compliance
Lightning Source LLC
Chambersburg PA
CBHW051613250726
48653CB00004BA/1486